Wrong Place, Wrong Time

WRONG PLACE, WRONG TIME

Trauma and Violence in the Lives of Young Black Men

John A. Rich, M.D., M.P.H.

THE JOHNS HOPKINS UNIVERSITY PRESS   Baltimore

© 2009 The Johns Hopkins University Press
All rights reserved. Published 2009
Printed in the United States of America on acid-free paper
9 8 7 6 5 4 3 2 1

The Johns Hopkins University Press
2715 North Charles Street
Baltimore, Maryland 21218-4363
www.press.jhu.edu

Library of Congress Cataloging-in-Publication Data

Rich, John A., 1958–
    Wrong place, wrong time : trauma and violence in the lives of young black men /
John A. Rich.
        p. cm.
    Includes bibliographical references.
    ISBN-13: 978-0-8018-9363-6 (hbk. : alk. paper)
    ISBN-10: 0-8018-9363-1 (hbk. : alk. paper)
    1. African American young men—Violence against—United States.
2. Victims of violent crime—Care—United States. 3. Youth and violence—
United States. 4. African American young men—United States—Social conditions.
5. African American young men—United States—Psychology. I. Title.
    E185.86.R52 2009
    305.38'896073—dc22   2009007046

A catalog record for this book is available from the British Library.

*Special discounts are available for bulk purchases of this book. For more information,
please contact Special Sales at 410-516-6936 or specialsales@press.jhu.edu.*

The Johns Hopkins University Press uses environmentally friendly book materials,
including recycled text paper that is composed of at least 30 percent post-consumer
waste, whenever possible. All of our book papers are acid-free, and our jackets and
covers are printed on paper with recycled content.

To Jessie and Fred, Nora and Theodore—
for keeping us safe and showing us how to live

Contents

Preface

Sadly, in many ways violence has come to define the urban neighborhoods of our country. African American communities especially have been tagged with the label of "dangerous" largely because of the young men who have become symbols of violence and crime. Violence remains a pervasive problem in the United States. Numbers tell only a part of this sobering story.

According to statistics from the Centers for Disease Control and Prevention (CDC), young black men have a higher rate of both fatal and nonfatal violence than any other group. National statistics show that homicide is the leading cause of death for African American men between the ages of 15 and 34. In 2006, 2,946 black males between the ages of 15 and 24 were victims of homicide. This means that the homicide rate for black males aged 15 to 24 was 92 in 100,000. For white males in the same age range, the homicide rate was 4.7 in 100,000. In other words, the homicide death rate was more than 19 times higher for young black men than young white men.*

Homicide numbers across the nation have decreased over the past decade, but a closer look at these homicide statistics shows disturbing trends. Daniel Webster and his colleagues at the Johns Hopkins School of Public Health have found that al-

*Centers for Disease Control and Prevention, National Center for Injury Prevention and Control, WISQARS (Web-based Injury Statistics Query and Reporting System), www.cdc.gov/injury/wisqars (accessed July 12, 2009).

though overall homicide rates have appeared stable since 1999, the homicide rate among African American men between the ages of 25 and 44 has increased substantially.* It is no wonder, then, that as these homicides are reported in the news, flashed across television screens, and recapitulated in films, we would come to associate young black men with homicide.

But homicide represents only the tip of the iceberg with regard to violence. Nonfatal injuries are far more common than fatal injuries. The CDC estimates that for every homicide, there are more than 94 nonfatal violent incidents.† Even with the increasing lethality of the guns available, the ratio of firearm-related injuries from nonfatal physical assaults to firearm-related homicides was four to one. In other words, for every person who gets shot and dies, another four get shot and survive.

While it is true that a person is more likely to die of a gunshot wound than from injuries delivered by other kinds of weapons, many young people are stabbed or assaulted. The ratios of nonfatal to fatal injuries for other types of violence show the same pattern. For those who are stabbed or cut, 64 people survive for each person who dies. For physical assaults, 3,243 people survive for each person who dies. In nonfatal injury, just as in homicide, black males are disproportionately affected. In data from the year 2000, the overall violent assault rate for black males was 4.6 times higher than the rate for non-Hispanic white males.‡ Countless others suffer trauma or near-trauma that never comes to the attention of the health care system, like being shot at or being grazed by a bullet or beaten up but not badly enough to seek medical care.

* G. Hu, D. Webster, and S. Baker, "Hidden homicide increases in the USA, 1999–2005," *Journal of Urban Health: Bulletin of the New York Academy of Medicine* (2008) 85(4): pp. 597–606.
† "Nonfatal physical assault–related injuries treated in hospital emergency departments—United States, 2000," Centers for Disease Control and Prevention, Atlanta, Georgia, 2002, pp. 460–63.
‡ Ibid.

Studies also show that violence is a recurrent problem. Up to 45 percent of people who have had a penetrating injury—a gunshot or stab wound—will have another similar injury within five years.* More disturbing is the finding that five years after their initial injury, 20 percent of these individuals are dead. Researchers have tried to identify predictors that will tell us who is most likely to be shot or stabbed again. Among the factors that predict reinjury are: being black, being male, being poor, past or current drug use, carrying a weapon, living in an unsafe neighborhood, unemployment, and prior arrest.† This research sheds some light on who is most at risk, but the risks are so general that they are associated with health risks other than violence and tell us little about how violence recurs. One study, by Carnell Cooper, a Baltimore trauma surgeon, mentioned the finding that several young black men cited "being dissed" as a cause of their injuries, hinting at more complex factors in the environment that might spur violence to erupt.‡

These young men suffer the full range of physical injuries, from the most severe, which result in hospitalization and severe disability, to the least severe, which are often cared for in the home by family or friends and never make it to an emergency department. Many recover physically, but the deeper and more persistent psychological wounds are often over-

---

* W. A. Goins, J. Thompson, and C. Simpkins, "Recurrent intentional injury," *Journal of the National Medical Association* (1992) 84(5): pp. 431–35; and D. W. Sims et al., "Urban trauma: A chronic recurrent disease," *Journal of Trauma* (1989) 29(7): pp. 940–47.

† See C. Cooper et al., "Repeat victims of violence: Report of a large concurrent case-control study," *Archives of Surgery* (2000) 135(7): pp. 837–43; M. D. Dowd et al., "Hospitalizations for injury in New Zealand: Prior injury as a risk factor for assaultive injury," *American Journal of Public Health* (1996) 86(7): pp. 929–34; N. S. Redeker et al., "Risk factors of adolescent and young adult trauma victims," *American Journal of Critical Care* (1995) 4(5): pp. 370–78; R. S. Smith et al., "Recidivism in an urban trauma center," *Archives of Surgery* (1992) 127(6): pp. 668–70; and M. G. Tellez et al., "Risks, costs, and the expected complication of re-injury," *American Journal of Surgery* (1995) 170(6): pp. 660–63, discussion p. 664.

‡ Cooper et al., "Repeat victims of violence."

looked. Even though large numbers of young African American men have suffered from violent injury, little research attention has been paid to the impact of post-traumatic stress disorder and other trauma-related symptoms on the lives of these young men. Because of this vacuum, we are left to rely on the vast store of knowledge gathered from military studies of combat veterans and studies of female victims of sexual violence or intimate partner violence. The key findings from this research are relevant to the circumstances of young African American men in the inner city, and they imply that we have underestimated the impact that violence has on these young men and their communities.

The Increasing Awareness of Trauma

In her seminal work *Trauma and Recovery*, Judith Herman eloquently made the case for the broad and penetrating effects of trauma, citing scientific knowledge acquired from studies on combat veterans and female survivors of sexual violence. She did not focus on inner city violence in young men, but many of her insights are relevant to this population. She cites studies of young combat recruits which show their vulnerability: "Predictably, those who are already disempowered or disconnected from others are most at risk. For example, the younger, less well-educated soldiers sent to Vietnam were more likely to be exposed to extreme war experiences. They were also more likely to have few social supports on their return home and were less likely to talk about their war experiences with friends or family. Not surprisingly, these men were at high risk for developing post traumatic stress disorder."*

Herman suggests that traumatized soldiers or rape victims are known to show symptoms of hypervigilance, which leave them constantly feeling as though they are in danger. Others are

---

*J. Herman, *Trauma and Recovery: The Aftermath of Violence—From Domestic Abuse to Political Terror* (New York: Basic Books, 1992), p. 290.

left unable to feel at all, which may lead them to subject themselves to danger in an effort to feel anything at all. Others return to danger to prove to themselves that they have mastered their fears. Others turn to alcohol or drugs to ease their pain.

Herman details with care how memory is disrupted in victims of trauma. They are unable to remember their traumas because the memories, shaped as they were by fear, were recorded without words, only with images; this is called traumatic memory. Even more important, she highlights the constant struggle that these individuals must engage in to find some meaning in their violence and to break loose from shame and guilt. Often they feel ashamed that they were so helpless in the face of danger and that they failed to resist or fight. Sometimes the shame of rape survivors is intensified by the implication that they brought the violence on themselves through their own actions—such as walking down a dark street. Combat veterans, Herman notes, are often left with the guilt that they could not save a friend or comrade. This survivor guilt can haunt them throughout their lives, even though they were powerless to save their comrades—or, in a sense, themselves.

These profound revelations about trauma, though harvested from the traumatic lives of women who have been sexually assaulted and soldiers who return from mortal combat, are important to keep in mind when we consider the social consequences of violence for the young men whose lives are detailed in this book. That so little has been written about their experiences is curious, since young black men are so often injured and reports of such urban violence dominate the news.

Broader Social Effects of Violence

It seems that the human cost of violence does not often get our attention as a nation. The financial costs, however, could. Costs of these various forms of violence are difficult to assess. Nevertheless, researchers from the CDC have reached the following conclusions:

- Americans suffer 16,800 homicides and 2.2 million medically treated injuries due to interpersonal violence annually, at a cost of $37 billion ($33 billion in productivity losses, $4 billion in medical treatment).
- People aged 15 to 44 years constitute 44 percent of the population but account for nearly 75 percent of injuries and 83 percent of costs due to interpersonal violence.
- The average cost per homicide is $1.3 million in lost productivity and $4,906 in medical costs.
- The average cost per case for a nonfatal assault resulting in hospitalization is $57,209 in lost productivity and $24,353 in medical costs.[*]

Phaedra Corso and her colleagues point out that, beyond the staggering human and financial costs of urban violence, violence in communities has broader social effects. They cite evidence that higher rates of post-traumatic stress disorder, depression, anxiety, suicidal ideation, and substance abuse are found in communities bruised by violence. Violence in neighborhoods breeds fear, which hinders community members from coming to the aid of others in need. Violence in schools leads to increased absenteeism because children are afraid to go to school. School violence also increases behavioral problems in schools.[†]

Fragmentation of urban families, while often attributed to lack of responsibility on the part of the father, may have significant roots in trauma itself. We know that traumatized people can find it difficult to connect to loved ones and to feel. We also know that in the setting of poverty and lack of opportunity young men may find it difficult to fulfill their responsibilities, even if they desire to do so.

Even more important, as you will see detailed in the stories of the young men in this book, a high level of violence in their

---

[*] P. Corso et al., "Medical costs and productivity losses due to interpersonal and self-directed violence in the United States," *American Journal of Preventive Medicine* (2007) 32(6): pp. 474–82.
    [†] Ibid.

communities makes young men feel physically, psychologically, and socially unsafe. Physically, young men who have been shot, stabbed, or attacked fear that unless they arm themselves, someone else might attempt to harm them as they have been injured before. Psychologically, they are left with the hypervigilance and disruption that come from trauma. Socially, they have often been raised in communities where there is a shared idea that if you fail to defend yourself when challenged, you become a "sucker," which will lead other people, who now believe that you are weak, to take advantage of you. This idea, which takes on a life of its own in communities where young people feel threatened, is also spurred on by ideas about what it means to be a man and what it means to stand up for oneself. When taken to its ultimate conclusion, this deep need to feel safe can lead young people to take up arms and retaliate.

Faces behind the Facts

Behind the statistics and data, behind the observations of researchers like me and urban ethnographers like Elijah Anderson, are the young men themselves. Sadly, because of their social position and the legacy of violence, racism, and poverty into which they have been born, they have become, for many of us, strange icons of fear. Each time a shooting or a stabbing or an assault is reported in the news, the details obscure a young man with a story, a young man with real blood running through his veins. Without any access to their voices, we could easily formulate solutions that are out of sync with the realities of their lives and that would be ineffective or outright destructive. Without hearing their stories, we lose sight of the young men who hold real hope for the future, whose visions for community embrace peace and nonviolence. This is why hearing their stories told through their own words is important. Not only does it reaffirm their basic humanity, it also points to a need to consider a different palette of approaches to violence and poverty and masculinity and nonviolence that might eventually yield enduring results for change.

■ ■ ■

I have chosen to title this book *Wrong Place, Wrong Time* because a similar phrase is commonly spoken by injured young men struggling to uncover the meaning behind their trauma. It is a perplexing expression, since many of these young people were not in the "wrong place." Rather, they were in their own neighborhoods, and they were often engaged in their usual activities—playing basketball, hanging at a night club or visiting friends in the projects. I believe that when they say "I guess I was in the wrong place at the wrong time," they are reflecting on the randomness of violence. They are asking rhetorically "What if I had left home 10 minutes earlier, like I was planning to?" or "What if I had taken a different street?" This kind of reflection is normal for traumatized people who are desperately trying to rewrite the script that led them to violence.

This expression should not be taken as subtle assignment of blame, as is often the case when the phrase is quoted in newspapers or television news reports. A deeper interpretation, from my perspective, is that the "wrong place" is a community abandoned and divested of the financial and human resources that are needed for community residents to remain safe. The "wrong time" might reflect a political environment that can only see these young men as "sick" or "bad" rather than "injured." Or that can only see punishment, rather than healing, as the single remedy for violence.

I add this caveat: there are some young men, both black and white, whose response to threat is shaped by a deeper mental illness—sociopathy, thought disorders, psychoses, or extreme addictions—and who do not and cannot hold this hope and desire for peace. But these young men are equally likely to be black as white. Some of their extreme illness has its roots in unimaginable early life trauma. The stories of these men are not represented here, but their need for treatment and healing cannot be overstated.

The stories recounted here convince me that there is a right place and a right time to understand how violence affects the lives of young men of color. The right place is the community, defined not simply by the neighborhoods where these men live but also the larger community of which all of us are residents. Now is the right time to hear the clear resonance of their voices and involve them as central participants in formulating the solutions.

Wrong Place, Wrong Time

INTRODUCTION

I will never forget the day in 1990 that I ran into my friend Dr. Jonathan Woodson in the stairwell at Boston City Hospital. Jonathan is a surgeon whom I first met when we were two of a handful of black residents training at the prestigious Massachusetts General Hospital. We both loved "The General," but, independently, we were both drawn to Boston City Hospital, a legendary public hospital famous for its care of poor patients and patients of color. We each chose to join the staff there—he as a trauma surgeon and I as a primary care doctor.

As usual, Jonathan wore a suit, tie, and a crisp white coat. He carried himself with the erect posture of the army reservist that he was. But this particular morning he looked unusually tired.

"We have to do something," he told me. "This violence is out of control. A couple of months ago, a young guy comes in with a bullet hole in his chest. We get him to the operating room in time. If that bullet had been 2 inches to the right, it would have gone straight through his heart. There are some tense moments, but we are able to do the repair. Save his life.

"Then this morning, I am driving to work and I hear his name on the radio. This same guy who we saved has been shot again. Only this time he's dead." He shook his head. "We have to do something."

Boston was in the midst of a bloody summer, and on many nights the emergency room brimmed with injured patients. Half of the beds on the surgical ward were filled with young men with gunshot or stab wounds. Nurses and social workers tried to care for each of them, but the pace was demoralizing. Even in the Young Men's Health Clinic—the clinic I launched a year earlier to provide primary care to young men making the transition from pediatric care to adult care—patients who came in for routine physical exams lifted their shirts to reveal scars left by violence or by a surgeon's attempt to repair it. Most also concealed the deeper emotional scars left by trauma and abuse.

"What do you think we should do?" I asked him.

"I don't know. Something. Anything. These guys sit up here in the hospital for days recovering. They literally do nothing! They just lie there in the bed. Somebody needs to talk to them."

Young people were dying. Others were permanently crippled. Jonathan and I shared the deep frustration of treating these devastating injuries that were so preventable. As black men, each of us felt the pain of seeing our community's potential lost, sometimes forever. These men were our reflection. We felt connected to them. But painfully, we felt powerless to do anything about it.

My encounter with Jonathan left me troubled. What he and I knew from our experience was confirmed by the available data. But the question remained: Why? Why were these young men getting shot and stabbed repeatedly? What could we say to them or do to them to keep this from happening?

As I struggled with these questions, I realized that, in the back of my mind, I held the implicit assumption that these young men had control over whether they got injured or not. Realizing that this belief sat unexamined in my head, I was disappointed in myself. Early in my career as a physician, I had learned that it was useless to blame people for what happens to them. We—doctors and nurses—are often wrong when we assume that we know why people do what they do in their often chaotic lives. But in this case, I realized that my assumption was the same one held by the police, my medical colleagues, and indeed, most of the people I knew. Simply put: young black men don't just get shot, they get themselves shot.

The presumption that all injured young black men deserve what they get is simple but powerful. It summons up images of black ghetto gangsters warring over turf and drug trade. It suggests that these fallen young men are rarely innocent bystanders but rather willing soldiers in some vicious civil war in the urban jungle. This presumption is pervasive and seldom questioned. Doctors, nurses, EMTs, and social workers are not immune to the effects of this idea. Young black male patients are assumed to be guilty of something. But where did this stereotype come from? And more important, is it true?

My own experience as a physician did not support this image, and most of the young black patients I saw in the Young Men's Health Clinic did not fit this stereotype. Kari, for example, had been injured when he tried to resist a robber's attempt to steal his gold chain. Baron was stabbed in a fight with a former friend. David believed that he had been mistaken for someone else. Others told me that they had been stabbed over "something stupid" like an argument over money, a dispute with a girlfriend, or a threat to someone's sense of "respect."

There were some, a notable few, who admitted that they sold drugs or were "down with a gang." Jimmy acknowledged that he was a "hell-raiser" in the Franklin Hill Housing Development, where he had grown up. He told me that the word in the street was that the masked man who shot him was a former partner in a gang who had a dispute or "beef" with him. Years ago, Mark used to sell drugs and carry a gun but had left all of that behind to make a new life for himself. But even though he grew up in the most violent streets in Boston, Mark did not cherish the chaos that came with the street life. When he did sell drugs, he did so "only until I get on my feet" or "until I can get a job."

At the same time, the patients who came to the clinic brought the typical medical problems of late adolescence—acne, sexually transmitted diseases, teen fatherhood, and marijuana use—as well as the aftereffects of their injuries. Macho and guarded at first, this posturing melted away within the first few minutes of conversation. Their attitudes were not menacing or aggressive. Rather, they poured out their apprehensions, often while shedding tears, grateful for someone who would listen. Something did not fit. How could these be the same menacing criminals that the police targeted every day, that doctors dismissed as hoodlums?

It was against this backdrop that I felt compelled to hear what the young patients who filled the beds on the surgical wards had to say about violence from their own perspectives. Over the next year, I interviewed 20 young black men who lay injured in the hospital and began to understand the power of their stories. Eager to expand the work, I applied to the National Institutes of Health to fund more interviews and in 1997, I received a five-year grant from the National Institute of Mental Health of the National Institutes of Health to carry on with my research.

Over the years that have passed since my conversation with Jonathan, I spent hundreds of hours listening to injured young black men, trauma surgeons, emergency room physicians, nurses, and other health professionals. Because they generously shared their stories, I now have a deeper understanding of the complexly intertwined phenomena of urban violence, the lives of young black men, and the scarring effects of trauma.

Along the way, I learned more about how the experience of being shot, stabbed, or assaulted drove many of these young men back to violent injury, not through the pathways that we usually assume but through the hazy fog of trauma. I have shared insights from this work with colleagues by speaking about this at meetings and conferences and writing articles for medical and public health journals.

But even as I wrote and spoke, I was troubled. In lectures and articles, limits on time and space forced me to reduce these narratives to their most basic elements. Although I was able to describe how violence combines with the social context to produce more violence, the voices of the young men got lost in the process. Also lost was the important and unexpected story of how spending hours and days with these young men transformed me. At best, the story was incomplete. At worst, I feared that these abridged versions of their involved and textured stories would unintentionally reinforce the disturbing stereotypes that had led me to this work from the start.

All of these reasons led me to write this book. I hope that in these pages, the reader will find a more complete and human rendering of these young men enlightening. But I must emphasize that it is a rendering—my rendering. To respect and protect the privacy of the young men I spoke to, names have been changed, details altered, and timelines compressed. Despite these necessary changes, the essential truths of their accounts, as I heard them, have been preserved. I hope the reader will encounter the deep humanity of these patients, the complexity of their trauma, and the sprouting seeds of hope that carry them into the future.

1

KARI IN PAIN

The September morning was bright, and the Boston air held a crisp edge that confirmed that we had left summer behind. Before leaving for the hospital, I punched the switch on the coffeemaker and walked down the stairs of my Roxbury home to get the newspaper. I then sat at the dining room table, bathing myself in the warm sun, and sipped the thick, strong coffee in preparation for the day ahead.

It was my routine to sit and drink coffee as I scanned the Metro section of the *Boston Globe* to find out whether any young men had been shot or stabbed within the past day. This sometimes seemed a morbid task, but it was the only way I could think of to meet these patients and hear their stories. The paper was just a place to begin, but if I found nothing there, then a walk through the emergency room later in the morning would likely yield one or two young men whose injuries had occurred after the paper had gone to press or whose tragedies were not considered dramatic enough to report. I surveyed the paper with ambivalence. On the one hand, I was sickened by the near-daily shootings that killed or crippled young people in my neighborhood. These everyday tragedies motivated me to do the research I would need to understand it. On the other hand, news of a violent injury meant that there was another injured patient to include in my research. Learning of a shooting helped the research progress. Still, I had to reassure myself as I looked up and down the columns of print. "I don't make it happen," I told myself. "They'd get shot whether I was researching it or not."

It was of no use, I learned over time, to look at the front page or even the first section of the paper. Unless a group of black men had been shot or violence had spilled out into the street and injured someone else (generally assumed to be innocent), the shooting of a young black male was not news. Most often the story was nestled in the second section, tucked between the lottery results and a report about the usual deadlocks in the city council.

I thought back to the night before, when I'd taken a shortcut through the emergency room on my way home from the clinic. As I passed through, I saw my friend, Dr. Lenora Holloway, sitting hunched over a pile of papers. She flashed a small, troubled smile. She looked down at the forms in front of her and said with resignation, "This is one young man who is not going to make it to your clinic."

I recognized the form. It was the Massachusetts death certificate. It is a painful form to fill out, for all the obvious reasons. But each field must also be completed perfectly according to the instructions or an administrator will reject it and force you to fill it out again. Even using blue ink instead of black ink will get the form kicked back.

"What happened?" I asked her.

"Well, apparently this kid was standing at a bus stop on Dudley Street, and a group of guys pulled up in a car. They blew this kid away. We counted seven gunshot wounds, and he was pretty much dead when he got here, even though that's a short ambulance ride. We tried to revive him, but he was gone."

She turned her attention back to the form. She raised her modern black horn-rimmed glasses and set them against her short afro. I couldn't help but notice that she was a strikingly beautiful woman. I had known her since she stood out in her class at Harvard Medical School. Now that she was a second-year resident, her eyes looked less bright and she seemed weighed down by the tasks of the day. But she, like most of us, had learned how to bracket her pain and emotions to get the work done.

Overhead, a voice announced, "Level 1 trauma. Gunshot wound. ETA 5 minutes."

Lenora looked up at me and shook her head while simultaneously stacking the papers and pushing them aside. "See? It just doesn't stop." She got up and joined the team of doctors and nurses who paused from treating patients with ear infections, dislocated shoulders, and out-of-control high blood pressure. There was little conversation as the team made their way to the trauma room. They had rehearsed this routine many times in the past and were primed from the young man they had been unable to save. Once in the room, each person took up his or her preassigned position.

I stayed in the hallway while Lenora moved to the right side of the trauma table. She pulled on blue latex gloves and began readying a large needle and syringe that she would use to insert a central line. The other members of the team took their places as well. A nurse dressed in green scrubs stood at the left of the table and sorted through a cart that held vials of medication that might be needed to revive or sedate the patient. A large pair of shears hung from her belt. The position at the head of the table was reserved for the senior emergency resident, who took his place and began preparing the endotracheal tube that would be inserted into the patient's windpipe in the event that he was having trouble breathing. Other physicians and nurses stood in their places, preparing the various tubes and medications that were always a part of the resuscitation routine.

The table itself was perfectly prepared, with a crisp white sheet folded across it. Bags full of saline hung in place, and IV tubing draped down on either side. A large cluster of intensely bright lights hung overhead, making the room look like an operating room.

Over a loudspeaker, a different voice announced, "Trauma 1. One minute."

I looked to my left and saw an ambulance backing up to the sliding glass doors. The emergency medical technicians and paramedics unloaded the patient from the truck by pulling on the gurney and allowing the wheels to spring automatically from beneath the moveable bed. One of them was holding an IV bag while the other pushed the stretcher from the foot end. They rolled the bed through the automatic doors, where they were greeted by a nurse who listened to their quick description and walked briskly with them down the hall toward the trauma bay, where the trauma team waited.

On the stretcher, a dark-skinned man who looked to be about 20 years old rolled his head back and forth moaning through the oxygen mask covering his face. His eyes were wide open, terrified, glazed. A large plume of blood stained his oversized blue jeans. His pant legs were split cleanly up to the knee on both sides. A spotless Timberland boot hung off his left foot, but his right foot was covered only in a dirty white sock.

The nurse who was walking alongside the gurney leaned over and asked him in a loud voice, "What's your name?" The young man did not respond but continued to wag his head. Suddenly, he raised his shoulders off the stretcher, looking as if he was trying to get up. The nurse, pushing him down firmly with her hand on his shoulder, shouted, "I need you to lie down and cooperate with us."

"I'm cold," the young man said, garbling his words as if his mouth were full of stones. The nurse continued to move, businesslike, seeming not to have heard him.

The team of doctors, nurses, and technicians surged to the stretcher as it pulled up alongside the table. Each person grabbed a handle on the long narrow "back board" on which he was lying. The senior emergency resident shouted "OK, one, two, three!" and in synchrony, the team jerked the board and slid the young patient onto the table. The ambulance gurney was removed, and in a scene that has always reminded me of a pit stop at a motor speedway, the medical team descended upon the patient and began the sometimes gruesome work of saving his life.

The senior emergency resident placed his hands on either side of the man's neck and deftly slipped a foam collar around it to hold it steady. Simultaneously, the nurse to the resident's left pulled out her shears and finished the job that the paramedics had started. She cut off the patient's baggy jeans, boxers, and jersey and peeled them away, leaving him completely naked.

Once again the young man began to grunt and reared up off the table as if he were desperately trying to find something. A large male nurse stepped beside the table and pushed the patient's shoulders down to the bed. As soon as he touched the bed, the young man arched his back and made a loud retching noise. Suddenly, large clumps of blood spewed from his mouth and soared up and out over both sides of the table. The dark clots hung in the air as if suspended in slow motion. The large nurse restraining the young man had just enough time to react. He spun away and ducked so that the patient's blood splashed across the back of his scrubs.

"Did that get you?" the resident asked as he suctioned out the man's mouth with a clear plastic wand.

"I'm okay," the nurse responded, twisting to peer over his shoulder at the mess.

"I'm going to intubate him. Give him a sedative and paralytic." A nurse pulled two syringes preloaded with clear medications from the cart while the resident readied a lighted scope with a long silver metal tongue. The nurse injected the medications—one a powerful drug to induce a temporary paralysis, the other a sleep-inducing agent—into one of the IV tubes. The young man's body instantly went limp.

The large male nurse calmly placed a rubber mask over the young man's nose and mouth and began to squeeze the large oval bulb connected to it, forcing oxygen into the patient's lungs. He forcefully pumped the bag and watched the young man's chest rise with each squeeze. At the resident's cue, the nurse removed this apparatus—called an Ambu bag—and the resident leaned over the young man's now-flaccid body. He pulled back his jaw and inserted the long blade, designed to move his tongue out of the way and expose his vocal cords. He held the scope firmly and with his other hand slid the clear plastic breathing tube into the young man's trachea. The nurse returned with the Ambu bag, this time attaching it to the breathing tube. He pushed a few more breaths into the young man, watching to be sure that his chest was expanding, proof the tube was in the right place. Finally, he connected the tube to a ventilator. Rhythmically and easily, the patient's chest began to rise and fall, as the machine pushed oxygen into his lungs. The resident grabbed the stethoscope that was draped over his shoulders and popped in the earpieces. He leaned over and listened to each side of the patient's chest before announcing, "Good breath sounds on both sides," confirmation that the tube was properly positioned in the young man's trachea.

Once this was done and the patient was rendered completely immobile, an intense calm fell over the room. Lenora squinted with concentration as she swabbed iodine on the patient's chest just beneath his collarbone, preparing to insert a central line into the large subclavian vein in the patient's chest.

Another doctor surveyed the young man's body for wounds, calling out her findings to a nurse who recorded the details on a clipboard. Even from where I was standing several yards away, I could see the slight hole in his right abdomen that was oozing just a bit of maroon blood. With the help of several others, the nurse rolled the patient up onto his side to look for other wounds on his back. She seemed unsurprised to see a much larger wound beneath his right shoulderblade, evidence that the bullet had entered his front and exited his back. Yet another nurse prepared to place a lubricated tube—called a Foley catheter—through the opening in the patient's penis and into his bladder. Next, a technician rolled the large portable X-ray machine into the room and began to take films of the man's chest and abdomen. Lenora confirmed that her needle was in the patient's subclavian vein by pulling back on the syringe's plunger and seeing a flash of dark blood. She slid the large IV line—called a cordis—into the patient's shoulder and prepared to secure it in place.

Less than 30 minutes after the patient was rolled through the doors, he was ready to move to the operating room. The surgical chief resident, who had entered the room quietly during the chaotic drill, decided that surgery was the only way to explore and repair the bullet's damage. The team packed up the patient and wheeled him quickly out of the trauma room and toward the patient transport elevator. No longer naked but covered in a cream-colored flannel blanket, the young man remained motionless. His feet hung off the end of the stretcher and his ashen heels rocked with the motion of the gurney. I stood and watched as he disappeared through the automatic doors.

Having seen this orchestrated chaos a number of times before, I was coming to understand its logic. These emergency room providers were driven by a single goal: get the patient to the operating room as quickly as possible. To accomplish this goal, they followed a well-rehearsed set of protocols that have been proven to work. Their approach would have been the same no matter what type of trauma he had suffered. The same routine would have been invoked if this young man had been in a car accident, nearly drowned, or fallen from the roof of his house.

The principle that drives these actions is referred to as the "golden hour." It is widely believed among emergency medicine and trauma physicians that if a trauma patient like this young man can be assessed, stabilized, and transported to the operating room within 60 minutes of his injury, he has a much greater chance of surviving. While some dispute the evidence that led to the concept of the "golden hour," few can dispute the effect that it has had on trauma care. The treatment of trauma is arguably the most highly standardized and choreographed treatment in medicine. There is little room for variation or creativity in the process. As a result, every trauma patient gets the same assessment, the same tests. He could be the CEO of a Fortune 500 company or an escaped felon who had been shot by the police. The protocols, the treatment, the effort are the same.

Still, I had begun to believe that something different happened when the patient was a young black male. Several impressions struck me as I walked out of the emergency department to my car. The first was that in the rush to save this young man's life, very few words were spoken to him, and he said very few words in return. "I'm cold" were the only intelligible words that I could remember hearing the patient speak. But there was also a sense that in the minds of the doctors and nurses and EMTs, each of these young black males who were rolling through the emergency department at such a frightening rate was the same. With few words spoken, it was impossible to distinguish between a young high school student struck by a random bullet on his way to school and a hardened drug dealer shot in a gang war. The faces of my colleagues (and perhaps they could say the same about me) showed that we couldn't care about these things or make these distinctions for fear that somehow it would hinder our ability to do our jobs. But as I walked away, the image of this young black male propping himself up on the table, desperate to say something, stuck in my mind.

That image came back to me as I took another sip of coffee and read the following brief in the *Boston Globe*:

> A young boy looked back at the spot in front of 1 Smith Street, where an 18-year-old Boston man was shot in the back during an armed robbery at around 6 p.m., yesterday. The victim was taken to Boston City Hospital where he was in stable condition last night, police said. Police are looking for a suspect who stole a gold chain from the victim.

■ ■ ■

When I got to the hospital, I leafed through the patient log in the emergency room. I found only one patient, Kari Brooks, who came in the day before with a gunshot wound. I saw from the record that he was taken quickly to the operating room and then to the intensive care unit. I rode the elevator to the 8th floor intensive care unit, where I found him lying in the private, high-tech room with tubes pouring out of his body. The tube that ran out of his mouth was connected to a computerized ventilator that percolated regular whooshes of air into his lungs. The tube in his right nostril ran down his esophagus and into his stomach. It drained out all the secretions that his injured intestines could not handle. Two tubes, one in each side of his chest, were connected to bubbling water chambers. These tubes, though painful and invasive, sucked out the bloody fluid and kept his bruised lungs from collapsing. Still another tube, a Foley catheter, drained amber urine from his bladder.

He lay still, deeply sedated and covered with a white sheet that accentuated his ebony skin. It would have been difficult to tell if he was alive, were it not for the mechanical rising and lowering of his chest and the beeping from the heart monitor. I could tell by the lack of even a spontaneous twitch or grimace that he was being maintained on a powerful paralytic agent, like the one that was delivered to the patient in the emergency room. The drug allowed the ventilator to give the patient oxygen effectively. But it also required that the patient receive potent sedatives, lest he be conscious and paralyzed at the same time, unable to let anyone know of his condition. I wondered if he was fully sedated or whether he could sense my presence at the side of the bed.

(I have heard stories from patients who were treated with these same paralytic agents but did not receive enough sedative to put them to sleep. For them, the effect was to be fully awake and to be able to hear providers talk about them in full candor, without realizing that the patient could hear them. They heard the voices of family members talking to them but could not achieve something as simple as opening their eyes or shedding a tear. For them, the effect was like that of being buried alive, full awareness of the fear, pain, and emotion swirling around them but unable to speak or respond.)

A nurse stood by his side, her back to the plate glass doors, and recorded his blood pressure, pulse, and other vital signs onto a blue chart. When I asked how he was doing, she said simply, "Fine. He'll make it." Then she paused, tilted her head to the side, rolled her eyes, and added, "This time."

I asked her, "What do you mean?"

She sighed. "It's like there's a revolving door out there. We take care of a few of these guys every week. And you can be sure that this guy or one of the others will be back again. Until they change their ways, it's going to keep happening."

"Oh, do you know how he got shot?"

"It's all the same. They say they weren't doing a thing. Well if that's true, how come they all have the new clothes, the new phone and the jewelry? Don't get me started. You should see some of this stuff. It's all gangs and drugs. You can take that to the bank. I've been around here for 10 years. I've seen it all," she said with a disgusted chuckle.

I didn't say anything in response, because I felt a deep ambivalence about the opinion that this nurse was stating as truth. I must admit that at one time, several years earlier, I would have agreed with her, perhaps even spoken the same words. But over the previous year, working with many young men in my clinic, I had developed an ambivalence that was difficult to articulate. Certainly, in the early 1990s Boston experienced a devastating epidemic of violence, where daily shootings resulted in two or three murders a week. Most of the dead were young black men. Most of them were killed by other young black men. Every day, I was faced with television and newspaper reports that made all young black urban men out to be gangsters or drug dealers or, worse, monsters or beasts. In fact, Mike Barnicle, a columnist for the *Boston Globe* newspaper began to use the word "beast" in his descriptions of young black men accused of committing murders in Boston. He wrote, "The case of the dead policeman momentarily exposes the public to a few of these beasts, and I use that word after consultation with Webster's, which defines predator as 'a plunderer, a hunter. One that preys, destroys or devours. An animal.'" Later in the same column, in defending his use of the term, he wrote, "Somehow, I don't think these people—the hard-working, God-fearing taxpayers of Roxbury, Mattapan and Dorchester—are going to be offended when words like 'beast' are applied to people who walk into an apartment and shoot two women in front of a baby. Here, words don't hurt, guns do."

It was hard to disagree with such strong language when applied to people who had allegedly killed police officers or unarmed women. But my discomfort grew when Barnicle and other writers so quickly threw this dehumanizing cloak over all young black men. He ended his column with these words:

> These kids are not going to grow up to be Colin Powell. They will not be Michael Jordan, either, or some other warm black male role model who make whites feel good about themselves.
>
> They are going to be our worst nightmare: an army of sociopaths who are a threat to themselves, to those closest to them and, inevitably, to the richer, white world beyond the borders of their miserable existence.
>
> You can kid yourself all you want or say it is racist to even discuss these things. But it is out there, percolating in a place most never see, where too many learn too fast to wake up each day angry, violent, with no conscience and quite ready to do business.

I hated this language. It offended me because of the way it labeled these very human young men to whom I talked every day. But I also took it personally. Somehow these verbal jabs aimed at young black males swung in my direction as well, as a black man. This was not because I recognized myself anywhere in the language that spoke about perpetrating violence. Rather, it was because all of these words, when aimed at the few among us, did violence to the rest of us.

But a stark reality remained: my colleagues and, to be honest, most everyone else I knew, we all carried around inside us an unspoken assumption. When a young black man rolled into the emergency room with a gunshot wound, we all assumed that it wasn't just bad luck. He didn't just get shot; he got himself shot. This assumption was confirmed in the murmurs that followed the patient's departure from the trauma suite. The ER team cleaned themselves up and washed their hands with a kind of disgusted satisfaction. Sure, they did their job and saved a life. But they were pretty sure, lacking evidence or information to the contrary, that they had saved the life of a drug dealer, gangbanger, or some other stereotype of a young black male absorbed from the news or television. They were desperate to stop this flow of injury and death, but there was a hovering nihilism that "these people" were who they were and nothing could be done about it. The nurse caring for Kari Brooks in the ICU was painting with the same broad brush, based on her own experience of seeing the most violently injured patients. But her impressions had to have been shaped by the reports that came up from the emergency room and by the opinions of providers who had little direct contact with young men like Kari. I was sure that her opinions had not been shaped by Kari because, in his paralysis, he was unable to utter a word.

After just two days, Kari was transferred to the regular surgical floor, and I made my way over to the surgical floor to see him. When I found him, he was awake, lying on his back in the bed. He did not move when I approached his bed, only turned his eyes toward me as if the rest of his body could not respond. Beads of sweat glistened on his forehead. He was no longer connected to a breathing machine, but he still had a tube in his nose and the double chest tubes that kept his injured lungs inflated. His breathing was heavy.

He asked, "Are you the doctor that will be here overnight tonight?" His voice sounded desperate.

"No, I'm not one of the surgery doctors. What do you need?"

"I was hurting a lot last night, all night long. I kept asking the nurses to give me something, but they said they had to talk to the doctor first. But nobody ever came, and the pain medicine they was givin' me didn't do nothin'."

"Let me talk to the nurses. I will see what I can do."

"Please," he stressed.

I started toward the door. Just then, Kari's mother walked in, followed closely by a short, thin man in sunglasses. She was a dark, stocky woman with short hair streaked with silver. She lifted her sunglasses and propped them on her forehead to reveal severe eyes rimmed by dark circles. Her brow showed creases of age that were inconsistent with her otherwise young-looking smooth skin.

"I'm Kari's mother. Who are you? Are you his doctor?" she asked with a tinge of annoyance in her voice.

"No, I'm not," I answered, "but I am a doctor here in the hospital."

"Well, who's gonna deal with all his pain? He's just laying here suffering."

"I can talk to his nurses and his surgeons and tell them that he is not getting relief." But even as I said this, I knew that my influence was limited. While I could advocate for Kari, I could not be sure that the doctors and nurses taking care of him would indeed be able to make him completely comfortable. Nonetheless, this simple reassurance softened her tone.

She did not introduce the man who was with her and who leaned warily against the wall behind her. He kept his sunglasses on and his head bowed, so it was difficult to tell if he was looking at me as I spoke, or at the floor. He seemed hunched and frail. I did not assume, since he had said nothing, that he was related to Kari.

Kari simply lay in the bed, looking increasingly uncomfortable. His mother looked toward him, and her face softened from anger to concern. "I would appreciate anything you can do. I hate to see him like this."

"Let me talk to the nurse," I said. I went to the nurses' desk and spotted a nurse named Debra who was familiar to me from past patients. She had always been kind and helpful, so I approached her.

"Are you taking care of the patient in 434?" I asked. She pulled a small square of paper from her pocket and looked at her list.

"No, he's not mine." She scanned the white board that hung over the nurses' station. "Jenna is his nurse." She looked up at the clock. "She's at dinner. Is there something he needs?"

"His family's upset because he was in pain most of the night, and he looks like he's in pain now. Do you think someone can get the on-call resident to take a look at him?"

"Poor thing. I'll go check on him now," she said before setting off down the hall. I felt better about leaving, confident that she would make something happen.

When I came by to see Kari the next day, his mother and an older woman were sitting in the waiting area. The older woman sat quietly on the couch, drumming her fingers on the large black purse that she held in her lap. His mother, who still looked trapped somewhere between worry and anger, paced slowly in the small area. Every few minutes she looked up at the lounge television that piped in a daytime courtroom reality show with the sound muted.

I greeted Kari's mother and asked if he had had a better night. "I don't know," she said with frustration. "We just got here but they are doing something to him, changing his dressings they say. They told us we have to wait out here, but it's been so long."

I nodded to the woman on the couch, and she nodded back. "That's Kari's grandmother," Kari's mother told me. She turned to the woman, "This is the doctor." She did all of this with little sign of interest, distracted either by the television or the unknown procedure happening to her son.

When I got to his room, I could see why his family had been dispatched to the waiting area. Debra, the same nurse who had checked on Kari the day before, was leaning over his bed, speaking to him softly and preparing to change his bandages. She wore gloves and a paper mask. The bedside table was piled with boxes of gauze, long cotton swabs, and bottles of saline and iodine.

Kari was lying flat on the bed without a pillow. He looked exposed, no longer wrapped in the blue hospital gown but shirtless, with a sheet pulled up to his waist. He had placed a white pillowcase over his face so that he didn't have to look at the wound. He fidgeted on the bed as he negotiated with the nurse about how to remove the soiled dressings.

"It's going to hurt when you take out the packing. The doctors are rough. Try to do it easy," he begged.

She answered sympathetically in a pleasant, low voice. "I will. You just relax and we'll go nice and slow."

She turned and looked at me, her blue eyes the only part of her face visible behind the mask and goggles. "He's got a pretty big wound," she said. "We're trying to clean it up."

I moved around to the head of the bed and lifted a corner of the pillowcase that covered Kari's face. He squinted up at me. "Hey man. Squeeze my hand if it helps," I told him.

Kari nodded and said "Okay." He gripped my hand and squeezed with surprising strength. I propped my other hand on the top of his head, letting it rest on the matted braids in his hair.

I offered my hand in a reflex that I pondered once Kari had encircled my hand in his. The hand squeeze is something I learned not in medical school but in the dental chair in my father's office. Sometimes, late in the evening after he had seen all of his paying patients, my father would sit me in the chair and begin the hour-long task of convincing me to let him numb my mouth and fill the cavity that had gone untreated for months. He and I would wrangle about whether to do it tonight or put it off until some later date. In the end, he would gently

convince me, but only after agreeing to let me squeeze his hand
while he injected the novocaine deep into my cheek. This was
a generous offer, since the hand that I would be squeezing was
the same one that he was using to separate my cheek from the
narrow gap between my tooth and the back of my mouth.
Though I was only 10 years old, I pushed all the power I had
into that small hand, taking full advantage of my father's offer
to share the pain when he didn't have to. But apart from that,
squeezing his hand helped to distract me not just from the ac-
tual pain but from the anticipated pain as well.

Kari continued to grip as the nurse removed the packing in
the deep wound and used sterile gauze to clean away the dead
tissue and infection. Even though she worked carefully, the exposed tissue was extremely sensitive. Kari clenched his teeth
and arched his back each time the gauze pad swiped the exposed flesh. He tightened his grip on my hand, doing everything in his power to follow Debra's instructions to stay still.

As I comforted him, I watched the nurse work and looked
down into the deep wound. It stretched from just below his
breastbone down across his belly, stopping just below his waist.

I was not trained to be a surgeon or to operate. But I often
saw wounds or skin ulcers on the limbs of my elderly patients
who had been confined to their beds for months. And I had
tended the shallow and stubborn ulcers that develop on the
young ankles of patients with sickle cell anemia. Usually the
sight of these wounds was not disturbing to me.

But here, standing in the bright and modern hospital room,
I began to feel queasy. It was not the stark red of the scant
blood on the discarded gauze or the pink white tissue in the
glistening wound that started to churn the space deep in my abdomen. These are sights that I had come to view as the normal,
even healthy appearance of the body trying to heal itself. But
something about looking into this particular gaping wound,
caused not by a chronic disease but by a bullet, and hearing
Kari's guttural moans of intense pain and feeling his desperate
damp grip on my hand pushed me out of the comfortable place

I normally occupied as a doctor. There was nothing to do. I considered slipping out into the hall, but then I thought about what it would mean to abandon this patient who was most in need of comfort at this moment. I steadied myself and forced myself to breathe, looking away from the gash and the instruments; I gazed instead out of the window, across the tops of the South End brownstones that framed the hospital in Worcester Square. After a moment, the odd sensation began to ebb, and after a moment, it had passed completely and I was able to focus again on what was happening before me.

The nurse continued her deliberate work. After a few grueling minutes for Kari, she had replaced the soiled packing with clean sterile gauze. She continued to talk quietly to Kari: "You're doing great, just a little more to do and we'll be done." He said nothing understandable during this time, offering only impatient sounds of fear and anticipation.

Finally, the nurse prepared for the last step of the procedure, which involved bringing the edges of the large wound together. She did this with a device that looked like an old-fashioned corset. Each side of the device was taped to one side of Kari's wound so that when it was gathered, it would bring together the edges of the wound. She prepared him for this step with a warning that held only enough information to make him squeeze my hand more firmly than at any other time.

"Okay," she said. "You are going to feel this. Just hold on." She performed this final maneuver quickly, and as she did, Kari arched his back and growled a high-pitched moan of intense pain. Small tears began to slide down his cheeks.

"Done," she said, quickly gathering the laces on the dressing to secure it in place.

Kari collapsed onto the bed and sighed.

"You did great, Kari," she told him, touching his arm. "I'll get you something for pain." She gathered the contaminated dressings with her gloved hands and blew a wisp of hair up off her damp forehead. She squinted a silent "thanks" at me from

behind the mask and hurried away. Meanwhile Kari lay pant-
ing and exhausted on the bed, looking up at me helplessly.

"You did well," I told him. "You're a trouper."

"I just want to get out of here," he said after a moment.
"Never wanna come back."

2

ROY IN PRERELEASE

As time went on, I got more and more frustrated with the constant newspaper reports of young black men being gunned down in the streets. The reality reached me every day in the hospital as well. As Jonathan and I encountered each other in the hospital hallways, our conversations would end with us both shaking our heads, unsure exactly what we should do.

I have to admit that I was also stung by a growing dialogue in the press, and even in the hospital, that black men like me were somehow to blame for all of the violence. The criticism was nuanced—and perhaps I was too sensitive to it—in bemoaning the fact that these misguided young men lacked mentors. I would often hear the opinion that there were no decent men in their communities whom they could look up to. Or it was sometimes said that all the positive men had picked up and moved their families away to the suburbs.

It was not just these conversations but also my own growing frustration that stirred my curiosity about what I could do, apart from my role as a doctor. Coincidentally, a friend told me about a newly funded mentoring program called the CLUB

(Career and Life United in Boston) that was being launched by the antipoverty agency in Boston for African American and Latino young men between the ages of 18 and 25. He told me that an orientation meeting was scheduled for the next night, and I agreed to go with him and learn about the program. Once there, I did not need to hear much more. They had the funding to provide educational support and mentoring for up to 50 young men, they told us. All they needed now were the mentors. Neither of us hesitated; we both signed on that evening.

Every Monday night, we would crowd into the small lobby of a nondescript building in the South End and sit in a circle. The topic for the night was chosen by Timothy Argenon, a bespectacled and earnest man who, though absent-minded and disorganized, had a unique ability to connect with young men from the many different worlds they came from. Early on, many of these young men were simply struggling. They were burdened and hindered by the poor schooling they had received in the Boston schools. Some had given up as early as ninth grade. Others finished high school only to find themselves with neither a clue nor a direction. Some were predictably plucked out of trouble just in time by a mother or brother who was able to prevail over them to find an alternative to the streets. As the program got more established, judges and probation officers began referring young men to it. Many of them were fathers, and as pressure mounted to take care of their children's expenses, they felt pressure to find a job or succumb to earning money in the streets however they could.

It was important for me to be at these meetings. The diversity of young men of color gave me a much-needed reality check and helped me reassure myself that I was neither crazy nor wrong. These men had lives that were as textured and complex as any of the patients I saw every day. Their struggles and their anger were counterbalanced by laughter and generosity. They were just as likely to open themselves up to talk about their past abuse and trauma as they were to boast about their sexual conquests. And, rarely, they were able to abandon their protective, hard, scowling expressions as their eyes filled with tears of which they were strangely unashamed.

It was at one of these meetings that I met Roy. I walked into the small computer lab housed in the agency building, and he was standing, looking over Timothy's shoulder at a computer screen. The intense look on his face bordered on anger. He stood defensively, with his arms folded across his chest, and only casually acknowledged me by turning his burning eyes in my direction when I walked into the room. I greeted Timothy, who was growing frustrated with some nagging computer glitch. "Damn," he said, not yet seeing me. I laughed, and he looked up. "Oh, hey, John," he said smiling. "This screen always gets stuck. So annoying."

Timothy turned toward Roy. "Roy Martin? This is Dr. John Rich. He was one of our first mentors here." Roy carefully held out his hand, but the scowl did not leave his face.

"Nice meeting you," I said.

"You too," he said.

Timothy excused himself, running off to connect with another one of the mentors making his way to the meeting. Roy and I were left standing there for a moment of awkward silence. Roy suddenly turned to me. "So what kind of doctor are you?"

"Primary care."

"Yeah? So what does that mean?"

"It means I take care of problems that adults have but I don't do surgery. I don't operate on people."

"What do you do, then?"

"You know, prescribe medications to treat diabetes, heart problems, skin problems. Pretty much anything that adults will get."

Roy nodded, seeming only partially satisfied by the answer. But I noticed that the stony look on his face had softened just slightly.

" 'Cause I got this problem right here." Roy lifted his cream-and-crimson striped polo shirt. He touched two fingers to his belly and ran them up and down the muscle just to the right of his navel. "Sometimes this hurts right here, and sometimes there's like a knot."

"Hmmm, a knot?" I asked.

"Yes. Here. Feel."

I felt odd about the request to examine his stomach in such a nonclinical place. Still, I said, "Sure. But let's just step out where there's not an audience." While we were talking, the computer room had filled up with other young men in the program, some of whom had looked up from their computer screens to take in the medical conversation. Roy shrugged and dropped his shirt.

"Don't matter to me. I'm cool with it." He scanned the other faces in the room, and his face hardened back to its original stone. We made our way between the closely spaced computer desks out of the room and across the hall, into a small classroom that was not in use for the usual English as a Second Language or General Educational Development class.

"Okay now, let me take a look," I said, sounding like I was seeing a patient in my clinic. Again, Roy raised his shirt. I bent slightly to look at the area. The skin looked normal. "I'm just going to see if I can feel what you feel there. Point again to the spot for me."

Roy again aimed his index finger at his belly. I followed his direction and felt the area with my fingers, pressing lightly and rolling my fingertips against the muscle.

"Don't feel anything like a knot there," I told him. "Can you feel it now?"

Roy placed his hand back onto his belly. "No, not now. But it comes and goes. The doctor out in Plymouth felt it, but he wasn't really trying to do anything about it."

"Is that where you are from? Plymouth?"

"No, that's where I was locked up. I'm in Boston prerelease now," he told me matter-of-factly. "That's how I got hooked up here."

"How is it there?" I asked.

"Prerelease? Not as bad as jail. At least I have the chance to get out, do some positive things, see my family. It's like being on a longer leash." He laughed, and I laughed with him now, seeing his scowl finally melt away.

"So how long were you locked up?"

Roy seemed surprised that I would ask. "I was only gone like two years on a three-year plea. I coulda gotten paroled, but instead I decided just to wrap it all up, do all my time. Things are still kinda hot for me in my neighborhood. And the funny thing about it though? I didn't even do the crime."

I nodded. As if anticipating my skepticism, Roy said, "Don't get me wrong, I have done some stuff that could have got me locked up. But they didn't get me for that. The thing they got me for, I didn't even do."

Roy looked me straight in the eye, and I was convinced. His eyes emanated a blunt honesty that matched his words and his voice. Roy had a "don't give a damn" attitude that I would see again and again as we got to know each other. At first it seemed confrontational and daring, as if he were waiting for me to disagree with him so he could take up the challenge. But later, I would begin to see it as a reflection of his satisfaction with and confidence in himself. He seemed, at that time, resistant to judgment by others. In a way, as paradoxical as it might seem, I admired him immediately for what seemed like a total lack of shame.

By this time, Timothy was walking around gathering the young mentees and the older mentors, directing us to join the large circle where the evening session would take place. He spied us standing in the small classroom and waved us toward the group.

"About to start," he said, rushing past us.

"You should come check out the place," Roy said. "I can have visitors there much easier than I could down in Plymouth. We can talk more there if you want."

"That would be great. Where exactly is it?"

"Down by the old Boston State Hospital, off Morton." He paused and then said, as if the idea were making more sense to him, "Yeah, come by. You gotta see this place."

■ ■ ■

The prerelease sat on the grounds of a long-abandoned mental health center in Mattapan. The buildings that used to be the old Boston State Hospital were barely visible through and over the trees as I approached them from Blue Hill Avenue. But the buildings I could see looked both desolate and dangerous. I remembered several occasions when the police found dead bodies on this land. I could think of at least one murder that was said to have happened here.

I turned left through the rusty and chipped wrought iron gate. A simple gray and black sign announced "Boston Prerelease," but there was no guardhouse, no one to stop me or make sure I had a reason to be here. I drove about a quarter of a mile, down the dusty asphalt road lined with untrimmed weeds and waist-high cattail reeds, until I came upon a large gravel parking lot stretched in front of an imposing red brick building. Another sign, simpler in design even than the first, confirmed that this was Boston Prerelease.

The enormous three-story building looked like a dormitory on a deteriorating college campus. But as I got closer, it looked like what it really was—the ruins of some dark asylum from the early 1930s. The building was surrounded by low weeds that pushed through the granite pebbles scattered between the patches of baked tan earth. A broken asphalt sidewalk pointed the way to the structure. The paint around the windows was peeling loose. Window shades hung crooked and tilted.

Looking up from the lot, I saw that each window was in motion. The heads of men of all ages and races trailed in and out of view, crossing the ceiling light bulbs that burned even though there was still sunlight. This could have been a scene from any urban college campus. The seething energy held the same mix of expectation, impatience, and possibility. The place threw off a palpable pent-up vitality that felt simultaneously suppressed: this was, after all, confinement. My sense was that these men were straining against a virtual leash.

I walked toward the small group of men sitting on the steps outside, waiting to board a blue van emblazoned with a shield reading "Massachusetts Department of Corrections." Not dressed in any discernible uniform, the three of them—one black, one white, and one Latino—looked as though they were relaxing in their own neighborhoods. The sandy-haired white man, whose cheeks were peppered with red acne cysts, was smoking a cigarette and staring off toward the traffic noise that spilled over from Blue Hill Avenue. The Latino man bent to whisper a private joke into the ear of the black man. He threw his head back and laughed out loud while his friend huffed a single sound of laughter and smiled.

I nodded as I eased between them and up the stairs, but they ignored me. Inside, a large African American man sat behind the counter. "Yes?" he asked.

"I'm here to visit Roy Martin," I answered.

He turned to look at an inmate standing in the doorway to the left. "Roy here?" The inmate shrugged.

Just then Roy appeared behind the man in the doorway and, without smiling, stepped around him and walked directly to me. The man at the desk asked, "This your visitor?"

"Yeah," Roy replied.

The man directed me to sign the book and produce a photo ID. I pulled out my driver's license and placed the laminated card on the desk. He picked it up and, without looking at me, copied some numbers onto a sheet. "Sign this." The form verified that I understood that it was illegal to bring any contraband to prisoners and that there were several actions, which though perfectly legal at any other place, could get me arrested if I did them here. I signed it illegibly and handed it back. Roy, who had been standing by me silently, turned toward the doors, and I followed.

The grounds around the building were sparse, and a cracked

asphalt drive wrapped around the back. Roy and I began to walk, automatically following the path. Roy let me know that while there was an air of freedom there, there were limits.

"We can walk around here as long as we stay pretty much on the property. I can only leave here to look for a job, see my family, and then go to the CLUB program. And then I gotta get signatures to prove where I've been.

"Everything you do here, they're just looking for a reason to send you back 'cause you messed up. But I definitely ain't tryna mess up. I try to stay out of my old neighborhood," Roy told me. "It's hard because I love my hood, and I love my homeboys. So I'd have a tough time separating myself from whatever was the drama of the moment if I was around all the time. Plus, I'll always have a family member on some wild shit, so the only places I go are to the CLUB program, to see my kids, and then to work and back to the prerelease. That's pretty much it.

"To tell you the truth, I could have got out of here on parole, but I turned it down. I didn't want to be back out there livin' in the projects, like an alcoholic sitting in a bar trying not to drink. But things are just too hot now. So I turned parole down. I'm just gonna stay in here another year until I wrap the whole thing up. That way I won't have to answer to some parole officer once I'm back on the streets. I also don't have to worry about the cops fucking up my life, lugging me back to jail for pissing on the sidewalk or something else stupid."

We strolled around the center and headed out between the great red building and the access road. The back of the building was scarred and tattered. The windows on the side had more peel than paint.

"This place is a mess," I thought aloud.

"Yeah," Roy agreed. "They're building a new prerelease on the other side, down Morton Street. So they ain't doing nothing to this one anymore."

"They told you that?" I asked.

"Every day. Every time somebody says the shower ain't working or the rain is coming in through the corner of the room, they say it. Nobody here really cares, since it's not like this is our home. I hope to be out of here way before they move."

Usually when I met young men like Roy, I was wearing a white coat and stethoscope. In that setting, in the clinic, I was expected to ask questions, dig deep, offer my advice freely. After all, it was my spot, my truth, my world at that point. Sometimes in the clinic, in that small linoleum exam room, it felt like we used made-up rules that would seem foreign outside. I could assure patients that their private confessions about their health, families, past shames, and misdeeds would never go any further. I could offer advice about safe sex and healthy diet and ways to deal with crushing stress without ever knowing with any certainty whether the patient had taken any of the advice seriously.

Here, though, in the bushy outback of the Boston State Hospital grounds, I was away from the comfortable isolation of the clinic. Here, the rules were not mine, the turf was different. And another thing rang clear to me: Roy and I could not have been more different. I did not know much about his life. He grew up steeped in a life that I could not yet imagine, not because it was so awful necessarily but because it was simply not knowable to me.

"So Roy," I said. "What can I help you most with? How should we work together?"

Roy twisted his face. "Hey, I got no expectations really. I just want to hear whatever you got to say that could help me. That's it.

"You've your experiences like school and becoming a doctor and all that. I've had my experiences too, been through lots of stuff, like school and family and the gangster life. So we've both been through a lot."

He nodded to punctuate the observation.

"So, what was school like for you?" I asked.

"I always liked school. I was one of those Metco kids. They got me into Lincoln Sudbury High School out in the suburbs.

I did good there too. All the teachers told me I should be a teacher like them."

"Lincoln Sudbury?" I asked. "Where is that?"

"To the west. Like 45 minutes. And I used to be out there every morning like 6 o'clock, waitin' for the big yellow bus. Hot or cold, rain or shine." He turned to me. "So you're surprised I was a Metco kid, right?"

Metco was the program that bused inner-city Boston youth out to suburban high schools. Unlike the contentious forced busing that led to street riots in the 1970s, this program was not just about racial balance. It was designed to give academically talented young people, most of them African American, a chance to attend a high-quality school.

I shrugged. "A little bit, I guess. I don't know much about you."

"Well, it's the kind of thing you see somebody coming out of jail, and you just assume they had a hard time in school. Or maybe that they came up out of one of those schools where they send kids who get caught with a gun.

"I was a little bookworm when I was a kid. That's really all I wanted to do—sit up in my room and read books. My brother used to make fun of me all the time. He'd say, 'You little fuckin' faggot.' But I didn't really care, 'cause I could always fight. My mother made sure of that. We either had to be fighters out there or get beat down by her. She was tough.

"So anyway, I remember it like it was yesterday. I was in third grade. And me and this Indian kid, we were best friends. And anything the teacher would give us to do? We would kill it. Murder it. Ace it.

"So this one time, the teacher gave us our tests back, and me and him both got 100. He sat across the room and we were holdin' up our papers, showing each other what we got. So there was this other kid, this fat kid, who sat between us. And I looked over at his paper, and I seen this big red zero. I don't know why the teacher did that but we was like, 'Damn. You got a zero?' Just makin' fun of him. You know how mean kids can be.

"So the teacher decides that to punish us for making fun of this kid, that she's going to put us in fifth grade, just to show us what it would be like to struggle, I guess. So she gets together with the other teachers, and they do it. They put us into fifth grade. And I'll admit that it was rough for about a week, but then after that, we were murdering that too.

"So they called my mother and told her the whole story and that they needed to put me in a different school. So they end up sending me over to this school for gifted kids over in Jamaica Plain, the Seaver School. That was a blast. I was taking French, speaking French. They even took all of us to Canada so that we could speak it up there.

"I wasn't really raised a street kid. I had street parents, but they didn't raise us street. They were like unrefined righteous people. Hardcore on right and wrong, and real extreme when it came to addressing wrong. I didn't really get into the streets too heavy until I was 12 or 13, pretty much the summer after finishing the eighth grade, just before high school. Really, to tell you the truth, I learned about the street from my family."

"Explain that," I coaxed.

"Well, my moms and pops started having babies when they were 15, so they were just kids raising kids. Add to that, they were the neighborhood tough couple. Badass mother, badass father, for real. So they taught us early, 'If somebody messes with you and they're bigger than you, pick up a brick or a stick and bust their head wide open. And if any of you see one of your brothers in a fight, you better jump in.'

"And my pops was a big one for trying to end a fight quick. So for him, busting somebody's head open to start off the action was the way to do things."

"Really?"

"Hell yeah. And he taught it to me. I had bricks in my pocket my whole childhood, and I couldn't tell you how many heads I split open with them bricks. If I was with my brother, he would start it off, and then I'd jump in—the little skinny kid with the brick. Bam! My parents never had a problem with us crushing people. They expected us to. Just like them."

"How'd you feel about that?"

"What do you mean?" Roy asked.

"I just don't know how I'd feel hitting people with bricks upside the head."

"Well, to me, the whole point in fighting is to hurt the other person. If you think about it, there ain't no fair way to hurt anybody. So my thinking is, if you're trying to hurt me or any of my people, we might as well get the hurting over quick. Only stupid people believe in fair fights; there is no such thing. There is only hurting. So when it comes to hurt-sport, you better hurt the other person quick or else you'll be the one hurting. That's what my father taught me.

"So in the end, I just got to be the big man in the neighborhood. And it wasn't even all bad stuff either. Sometimes people depended on me to keep the peace too."

"You were like the police, huh?"

"I'm serious, man. Like there was this guy in the neighborhood who was goin' around robbin' people's mothers. So I found out about it, and I shot him in the butt. Suddenly, I was like the town hero. Mothers were sayin' to me, 'I'm sorry my punk-ass son didn't shoot him.'" Roy laughed at the thought.

"Is that what landed you in jail?" I asked.

"No man, that was like community service there. Nobody's gonna turn you in for that. Nah, I got locked up for something else.

"I had drama with some dudes from my neighborhood, dudes I grew up with; some of them were even from my own crew. But they had drama with one of my uncles, and they ended up shooting at each other.

"Now, I don't know what made them think it was possible to get into it with my uncle without me jumping in, 'cause I take all family issues seriously, especially if it's my own crew who's doing the violating.

"Basically, they robbed my uncle. So I told everybody, 'If my uncle doesn't have his shit back in a week, then y'all might as well "suit-up"'"—meaning, arm yourself for war.

"I don't really want to talk about the details, all I'll say is that the deadline came and went, and my uncle didn't get his shit back. So I did what I promised I'd do.

"I went to a certain person's house, while he was having some kind of family reunion or something. I showed up with two of my best gunners, and by the time the night was over, nine people were shot, and me and my two boys were locked up. That's what I'm doing time for. Weapons, the shootings. That's the case that got me here."

I strolled alongside Roy, nodding my head and squinting with interest. I had asked the question about how he got there without expecting this level of terrifying detail. As Roy spoke about his past life matter-of-factly, I wondered if I could really relate to Roy and address issues about which I knew so little. In my interactions with patients, I asked whether they had been to jail, but I rarely got the level of detail that Roy was giving me. Roy was giving the kind of information that most providers would rather not know.

"But I really didn't think I'd get convicted for the shooting, though, because these were tough guys, not cowards. I didn't think they'd snitch, since nobody died. I learned something though: tough ain't what tough used to be. They told the cops everything but used fake names either at the hospital or the police station.

"So I ended up going to court against names I didn't recognize and names that I know were made up. So I never thought anybody would show up to trial. How could they track down a fake name? So I figured they didn't really have a case against me."

Roy bent to pick up a granite pebble and lofted it out into the woods. "I didn't care about sitting in jail. Nobody was gonna beat me up in jail. All of the males in my family have done time. We all go to prison at some point. So it was no big deal to me.

"But I got nervous when the indictments just kept coming. And then weird witnesses started showing up, telling stories that were clearly fiction, but the court kept indicting me for shit.

"I guess it just got to the point where I was feeling like I had done so much bullshit out there that I was going to end up in prison for being *Roy*, not necessarily for doing this particular crime. Something was making sure I was going to prison, it was just a question of how long.

"Back then, Boston was sending brothers to jail for anything. With the record murder rate, there were lots of false murder convictions. I wanted to go to trial to at least force these washed-up tough guy niggas to snitch. But all I saw were niggas getting sentences of 14 to 20, 7 to 15, 15 to life.

"So I said, 'Fuck it.' I ain't even trying to beat this case, I'm just trying to get the best deal. I didn't want to go to trial and suddenly have one of these dope fiends show up, snitch, and walk free because he helped convict me. I could have gone away for a long time. My first offer was 27 to 45 years.

"But to everybody's surprise, I pleaded guilty. The judge gave me nine concurrent 3 to 5 year sentences for the shootings. So I took the deal and got 3 to 5 years."

I pondered what Roy told me as we walked. He took a plea because he wanted to avoid the chance of a longer sentence. It seemed to me that the things Roy did in the past had not netted him nearly the negative consequences they could have brought. He never got shot or stabbed or seriously injured. He served far less time in jail than he would have gotten had he elected to go to trial. I wondered then what motivation he had to change his life around.

It was clear that Roy was smart, even brilliant. He did not tell me the details of his street life, but I imagined that he had done well and that some of the wealth he had accrued might still be hidden away in the projects somewhere. In the past, it might have supported his friends and family and made him the man that he was in the community. And so, having suffered no consequences, what would make him give up his tough guy gang leader identity and focus on the small things that could make his life better?

So I asked, "What will be different this time when you get out of jail?"

Roy was quick to answer. "You said it right there: the fact that I've been in jail. When this is all done, I will have been away for three years. Away from my daughter. Not having the chance to see her grow up. Away from my son. That's what keeps me focused. I never wanna see the inside of the jail again. I don't care what it takes."

"Are you saying that jail has been a good thing for you?"

Roy twisted his face. "Well, yes and no. Yes, because I don't want to go back. No, because all that time wasted just made me angrier. I'm only 21. I already lost two years and looking at one more. And so the hardest part is to get over the anger of going there in the first place and the fact that so much of my life is gone. That's my problem to deal with."

3

JIMMY IN THE HOSPITAL

On Monday morning, I did my usual scan of the morning paper and found that over the weekend another young man had been shot in the Dorchester section of the city. The paper noted simply: "Shooting in Franklin Hill: Police were called to the housing development when residents reported gunfire. When they arrived they found a 17-year-old suffering from multiple gunshot wounds. The unidentified young black man was transported to Boston City Hospital. Police are investigating whether the shooting was gang or drug related."

I sighed as I read the last sentence. It seemed that every report of violence involving young black men carried this disclaimer. It was as if the reporters were trying to reassure readers that violence only happened to young men who were in gangs or who sold drugs. My own conversations with these young men had taught me that violence was more complex than gangs and drugs, and I wondered what my conversation with this young man would reveal.

At the hospital I found a listing in the emergency department log that matched the description of the young man in the paper. The name in the log read "Jimmy Parker." He had gone straight to the operating room and then to the intensive care unit for a day. Since he was only 17, Jimmy was then transferred to the pediatric adolescent ward. I made my way upstairs and passed through the usual tan and gray adult hospital ward decor. But when I passed through the doors to the children's ward, the decor changed to brightly colored walls adorned with cartoon images and balloons. The ceiling was painted sky blue and was dotted with happy cumulus clouds. In some of the rooms, children played on large portable video game consoles that the nurses shuttled from room to room. Children with sickle cell anemia, asthma, cystic fibrosis, and other chronic diseases occupied the rooms on this ward along with patients who had bones broken from falls or car accidents. Once in a while younger patients like Jimmy, who had almost been killed by gunfire, found themselves on the same ward.

As I approached Jimmy's room, a tall blond nurse dressed in a bright white pantsuit and spotless white clogs pulled me aside.

"Is that who you're coming to see?" she asked, pointing toward the corner room.

"Yes, why?" I asked.

"Well, I think he's in a gang. He stays on the phone talking to his friends. All he talks about are the streets and how he wants to get the people that did this. He doesn't care that I hear him. I tried to talk to him, but I don't think he gets it yet. You know what that means."

She looked at me with a furrowed brow, waiting for a response. Her steely blue eyes, carefully framed with perfect mascara, tightened with intensity, and she blinked deliberately.

She leaned a bit closer. "We'll see him again. I'm sure of it. And I really worry about him."

Her face radiated sincerity. Still, I didn't know what to say or think after this. Maybe since this was a pediatric ward, the nurses didn't see many young men this age with gunshot wounds. Perhaps she was just being extra careful. But as I walked the rest of the way to Jimmy's room, I wondered if she had formulated her own stereotype: all black men who got shot must be in a gang. The morning's newspaper report may have swayed her as well.

Still, over my ten or so years as a doctor, I had learned to trust the nurses' instincts. More than one attentive nurse had realized that a patient was starting to slip into heart failure long before I would have noticed on my twice-daily visits. This pediatric nurse spent hours in and around this young man and other patients just like him, a simple fact often lost on us doctors. She was his primary caretaker, so her worry was valuable information.

Yet standing at his door, I couldn't help but hope that she was wrong. The chubby patient propped up on the bed looked so young that it was a stretch to call him a man. He looked unusually short, and his body was wide and stocky. His round face sported baby-fat cheeks on smooth beige skin marked only by a small crusted wound on the left side of his face. His eyes were clear, bright, and brown with a hint of moisture at the corners. There was a trace of early stubble on his chin, and his hair was in fuzzy cornrows. A small hole in his left earlobe marked the usual location of an earring.

"Hi, my name is Dr. Rich. How are you feeling?"

" 'Bout as good as I can expect, I guess. I'm living though." He shrugged as if to offer all of his wounds to me for inspection. "Where you gonna poke me today?"

His speech was thick, and the left side of his face was puffy where the bullet had pierced his jaw. The bullet had cut through the nerve that controls his facial muscles and his left eyelid. When he blinked, his left eye closed only partially. When he tried to smile, only the right corner of his mouth responded. The rest of his face looked clumsy, as though it had been injected with novocaine. His arms were propped up on pillows, and a fiberglass cast encased his left arm.

"I am not one of the surgical doctors who are taking care of you. I am one of the primary care doctors here in the hospital, and I am talking to young men like you, trying to understand what it is like for a young man like you to get shot. I wonder if you would mind talking to me sometime in the next few days."

Jimmy looked up at me with a quizzical look on his face. "You want to interview me? You mean like a reporter?"

"Not exactly. But I want you to tell me your story. I mean, you have been through a lot, huh?"

"Yeah, man. Look at me," he said.

"And not just you, I bet, but your family too, huh?" I added.

Jimmy looked surprised for a moment and then lowered his head. His eyes welled up and tears began to run freely down his face. He shuddered once, trying to get control of the flow, but more tears came instead. I stepped to the bed and rested my hand on his heavily bandaged left arm.

"I just started thinkin' about my brothers and my sisters and how they was gonna be hurtin'. They love me a lot, a whole lot, and I love them. If I died, what would they do not being able to see me every day?" He turned and used his shoulder to rub away a tear.

"When I was lying there shot, I was just thinking, 'God, am I going to die on them like this?' I usually see them every morning, before I leave the house. But I didn't even see them that morning or nothing, you know what I'm saying?" He started to sob again.

Just then a tired-looking surgical resident appeared in the room to begin the meticulous daily inspection and cleaning of Jimmy's bullet wounds. Jimmy turned his head again to mop his eyes on the gown and wiped his nose with the back of his right wrist. He put his head back on the pillow and breathed, trying to collect himself.

"What, you again?" Jimmy teased, sniffing and half-smiling.

The resident flashed a wry grin. "Yep. Glad to see you too."

"I hope you not gonna be diggin' in these wounds again. That shit hurts, man. Didn't you do enough of that last night?"

"No digging, just looking," the surgeon answered while sorting through a bright blue case that looked like something made for carrying fishing tackle.

Jimmy was not reassured. "Well, you know I need some pain medicine before you do that."

"Looking doesn't hurt. No extra Percocet." The resident had stopped smiling. He pulled on blue latex gloves and moved to Jimmy's arm with a curved pair of scissors. Jimmy braced himself and turned away, anticipating pain.

I decided this was not the best time to continue our conversation. "I'll be back later," I told Jimmy.

"Okay," he replied. "What's your name again?"

"Here's my card." I tucked it into the drawer of the bedside table and turned to leave.

"Make sure you come back," he called after me.

"Don't worry, I will."

■ ■ ■

The next day, I found Jimmy sitting in the large gray recliner, carefully perched like a small prince on a throne. Each bandaged hand sat neatly on the arm of the chair, a soft white blanket draped perfectly over his legs. Jimmy lifted his head off the pillow when I walked in, but he did not smile. "Hey Doc," he said and laid his head back on the tall pillow.

"Do you feel like talking?" I asked.

"Yeah, I always like to talk. Even though I just got some bad news. The doctors are telling me my face might stay paralyzed like this. I hope it don't, but they say it could."

"We can talk later if you want."

"Nah, let's talk. Might give me something to do, something to make me feel better. I just can't talk too good 'cause of my face."

"That's fine, I can understand you."

For a moment, as I pulled up a chair, Jimmy turned and looked out of the large bay window to his right. I looked too. There was a spectacular view across the rooftops of the nearby brownstones, and in the distance I could see the metallic blue Hancock Tower.

He was still looking away when I asked him if he would tell

me how he got shot. Jimmy turned back and instantly engaged me as if I had startled him from a brief dream. "I was coming from my uncle's house, like 11 at night. I was over there taking my cousin's bike back, 'cause I had borrowed it. And when I came downstairs, this dude was just standing in the doorway with a gun. I think he had a .45. I didn't know who he was, you know what I'm saying? I mean, I know who he is now, because later, I kind of recognized him. But he just shot me in the face.

"I fell down, got back up, and just started running through the hallway trying to get out the other side of the building. And as I was running through the hallway, he was just chasing me, shooting me. He shot me five more times.

"Then he stopped, turned around, and ran out the other way that he came in. So I just ran out of the building and into another building, where I knew there was a lady with a phone in her house that I could get to.

"When I got up there, I banged on the door. She came to the door real quick, let me in, sat me in a chair. Then she called the ambulance. The person on the phone told her to put pressure to my bullet wound on my shoulder, and that's what she did. And like fifteen minutes later, the ambulance came and rushed me to the hospital. That was about it."

"How do you know who shot you?" I asked.

"Well, about an hour earlier, my cousins came running around the corner telling us that this dude and his boy was around there. We didn't think nothing of it."

"That didn't make you worried?"

"Nah, I wasn't worried about it because I know him. He used to be my crime partner, and I knew I didn't have no beef with him. I knew that he had problems with certain people around there, but the people that he had problems with weren't around. But come to find out, he wanted to do something to me too. He wanted to kill me."

"Over what?" I asked.

"I don't even know," Jimmy responded. "That's my whole point. But I really, really, really want to know why he did that.

I just want to get him face to face and ask, 'Why did you shoot me?' But I'm going to find out, though." He pointed his finger at me to underline his point.

I was distracted by Jimmy's revelation that he had a "crime partner." The same feeling of ambivalence came over me that I felt when I was scanning the papers for reports of shootings. I was worried for Jimmy but at the same time intrigued by what he might teach me. Up to this point, only a few young men had been willing to talk so freely about what had made them get involved with violence and crime. None of the other men who dared reveal this part of their lives were as young as Jimmy. But I had to part now with the notion that Jimmy was a misunderstood cherub.

His nurse was right. I remembered her cautions from the day before. Jimmy's childlike appearance and his tears of the day before had me thinking that this must have been a random act of violence. Propped up as he was in the chair, surrounded by heavenly images of clouds and hot air balloons, it seemed remarkable that he could be both child and gang member.

"Tell me about getting to the hospital. What was that like?" I asked.

"Oh, man, it was rough making it here." Jimmy leaned up in the chair, more animated as he realized there was so much more to tell. "The cops got there first. They came in the house and the detective was like 'Who shot you? Who shot you?'

"I'm like, 'I don't know.'

"He kept on saying it. 'Who shot you? Who shot you?'

"And I just told him again. 'I don't know.'

"Then the EMTs just put me on a stretcher, took me down two flights of stairs, and put me in an ambulance. Then the police came onto the ambulance and said it again. 'Jimmy, you got shot six times, man. You ain't going to make it. You're going to die. Who shot you? Who shot you?'

"So he's sitting up there saying it, and I know I've been shot six times, so I'm thinking I'm not going to make it either. So I'm like, 'Damn.'

"So the cop starts up again. 'Who shot you, Jimmy? Who shot you?'

"And I'm like, 'I don't know, man.'

"He's like 'C'mon, man, you ain't going to make it.' "

This time Jimmy's voice rose into an insistent nasal whine as he reenacted the chaotic scene.

"I'm like 'Man, I do not know who shot me.'

"So I say to the paramedics, 'Man I'm sittin' up here bleeding to death. Could you all take me to the hospital, please?' Then they were like, 'Yeah, we got to take him to the hospital. He's bleeding pretty bad.' "

He stopped for a minute, then a smile spread across the side of his face.

"What's funny?" I asked.

"Well, it wasn't funny then. But now it's funny. Actually it's kinda sick. But the ambulance dudes? They start arguing about where to take me." He shook his head.

"They was just like 'Which one should we take him to—the Brigham or City?'

"One of the paramedics was like, 'Let's take him to the Brigham.'

"I'm like, 'No, man, that's too far, you know what I'm saying? City's right around the corner, man, you know what I'm saying?'

"And the other one was like, 'Yeah, we should take him to City, since that's closer.' And they just brought me to City."

I chuckled too, but for a different reason. The crosstown hospital the Brigham and Women's Hospital enjoyed a worldwide reputation for excellence in medicine. In the poor neighborhoods of Boston, however, the word on the street was, "If I get shot, take me to City." What Boston City Hospital lacked in amenities, it made up for with its robust street reputation as the best trauma hospital in Boston.

Jimmy went on: "To be truthful, I thought I was going to die because my heart, I just felt it going slow. All that was running through my mind was 'I'm going to die, 17 years old.'

"As soon as I got to the ER, they picked me up and slid me onto the table. There was mad people in the room and these big lights. Then I felt them digging in one of my wounds, cutting off my clothes and uncovering my wounds. And then I was just asleep.

"When I woke up, I thought it was Wednesday. The doctors was like, 'No, it's Friday.' I was like, 'Whoa!' They was like, 'Yeah, you were unconscious for a couple of days. You lost a lot of blood. You almost didn't make it.' I was like, 'Whew! Thank God He kept me around.'" He sighed deeply, satisfied to have reached the end of his tale.

Jimmy did not wait for me to ask another question but leaped right in again: "But my family is deep. I mean we look out for each other. We all got the same mentality, my whole family. We ain't crazy but we all act the same, react the same, you know what I'm saying? It's just that everybody knows my family, man. Everybody."

"Tell me what you mean when you say you're all the same, you act the same," I asked.

"Like if my cousin was to get shot like I got shot, my whole family would be very upset. They would be dying to get their hands on him.

"That's how I like it. That's how I want it to be. I don't want them to just be like 'Oh, he got shot,' and they don't think nothing of it. Because I know if somebody shoot my family, and I know who it is, I'm going to try to get that nigga's head, you know? And that's how they think, too."

Jimmy continued to tell his stories in his own way, with a rough edge. There was not a hint in his voice that he was editing or deferring to me in any way. He was, it seemed, telling me not so much what he thought but how his life was. Because he was so clearly unfettered, I viewed him as an honest expert on what other young men had told me.

"Can I ask you about something that I've heard other young guys talk about?"

"What?"

"Can you tell me, what does it mean to be a sucker?"

"A sucker?" he repeated. He spit out a puff of air like I had asked him a question with an impossibly easy answer. "Not to stand up for yourself. A sucker means people pick on you. You know what I'm saying?"

I nodded, waiting for him to break it down for me. "Nowadays, there aren't too many suckers out there. There's a few but not too many."

"What do you mean?" I probed.

"It's like this: Everybody's trying to ill these days, everybody. It used to be the older brothers, but now, it's all the young niggas illin'. All the young niggas is trying to earn their stripes."

"Earn their stripes?" I parroted, a not-so-subtle prod for him to explain. I felt for a moment like the stiff police detectives of *Dragnet*, the police show that kept my sister and me pinned to the black-and-white RCA console television that sat at the foot of the basement stairs.

"Yeah, trying to make a rep for themselves, you know what I'm saying? That's what I did, running around busting mad caps."

"Busting mad caps?"

"Shootin' guns," he replied, matter-of-factly. "When I go up around my neighborhood, I'm known by everybody. Everybody knows me. That's why I don't get into beefs with too many people."

"So that's why young guys want to have a rep?"

"Yeah. So people can know them. Just to be known." Jimmy paused and pulled at a snag in the blanket that covered his legs. After he had tugged it until it would not yield any farther, the fabric bunched together into what looked like a small scar. "People don't like to be nobodies these days; they like to be somebody or try to be somebody."

"So, how do you get to be somebody?" I probed.

"You got to just put in work," he answered.

"What do you mean?" I asked.

Jimmy lifted the volume of his voice slightly. "Busting caps.

Busting heads. Whatever. Violence. You know what I'm saying? You got to *do* something. You got to *earn* it."

He locked his hazel eyes on me and repeated himself: "If you
want to earn some stripes or get a reputation, you got to *do
something* to get a reputation."

Jimmy slumped back into the chair as if he were tired of
teaching on this subject. But then he piped up again.

"You can get a reputation for doing good things too. Like if
I was talking to little kids, telling them what's right and what's
wrong, I could get a reputation for that too. People would say
'He's good now. He's chilling out. He ain't messing around.' "

He cocked his head to the side, as if he were weighing the al-
ternatives in his argument. "But then you still got some knuckle-
heads that don't care if you're doing good. If you did something
to them or to their people, they still want to get you, no matter
if you're doing good or not."

He looked off toward the bed and sighed heavily. I scanned
the room where he was staring. The room was most notable for
what it lacked. There were no get well cards with animated zoo
animals. No helium-filled mylar balloons proclaiming "We
love you!" or "Get well soon!" Only a gray and silver portable
Sony CD player hinted that someone had come to comfort
Jimmy or support his recovery.

"Who brought you the CD player?" I asked gently.

"Oh, my sister brought me that. She came up here yesterday."

"What about your mom?" I asked.

"I only seen my mom once here. She came up here while I
was still in the ICU. I couldn't talk because they had that tube
in my throat, so I just reached up with this hand and wrote 'I
LOVE YOU' on her chest. She just busted out in tears and ran
out the room. Later they told me that she went downstairs and
was raisin' hell, kicking stuff over and screaming. The security
police had to make her leave, and they told her she can't come
back here no more."

"It had to be really hard for her to see you like that," I said. I imagined the scene he described of a black woman screaming hysterically about her son. I had seen these moments a few times, most often in emergency rooms after a family had been told that their son was dead. Even then such displays were carefully controlled by the security guards so they did not spiral out of control.

I was reminded of the displays of grief that I have seen at black church funerals, especially those for tragic deaths, like the murder of a young man. I have witnessed whole families wailing, collapsing on one another and on the floor, stretching out over the coffin, begging the young man to get up, screaming, "Why? Why?" But these emotional church moments never spiral out of control, and never have I seen church ushers intervene in any way. The grief and wailing have their own rhythm and purpose there. Sometimes in the hospital, I have wondered if it wasn't the presence of security personnel, both visible and invisible, that causes chaos to erupt. Sometimes it is the preparation for chaos that beckons that very chaos into existence.

The hysterical display that Jimmy described was less often tolerated from the family members of patients who are still alive. But still, it was hard to imagine that Jimmy's mother was both escorted out of the building and banished from visiting ever again.

Jimmy interrupted my thoughts. "My mom's a good person, you know what I'm saying? She just has problems of her own. And she ain't just gonna break out of them on her own. She's gonna need help. She uses cocaine, so I know she ain't gonna just up and quit. I still love her, even though she do what she do. I love her to death."

"What about your father?" I asked.

"He's locked up now. But he should be getting out in a couple of months," Jimmy responded. "But we don't really got no good relationship. He was never there for us when we was growin' up. He came around sometimes, but he never did any kid stuff, never did nothing with me. Nothing. Absolutely nothing." Jimmy turned to peer again out of the large window. "I hate him for that, but I love him. I still talk to him, but he knows. He knows."

Jimmy reached down for the multicolor remote resting on his thigh and pressed the nurse call button.

"How are you doing?" I asked.

"Startin' to feel some pain, that's all. She usually brings the Percocet by now."

Within a minute, the same nurse that had greeted me the day before entered with a small white medicine cup. "I was just on my way," she said as she filled a pink plastic cup from the pink plastic pitcher of water on the tray table.

"Jean is my favorite nurse," Jimmy said in a voice that remained nasal but had now taken on a slightly flirtatious tone. "She's always on the case, right on time."

She said nothing but smiled and dumped the pills into his only good hand. She waited for him to put them in his mouth and then handed him the pink cup. Jimmy sipped several times, working to get the pills down. The nurse looked down at me knowingly, and I looked back up at her and shrugged with my eyes. She gave a slight nod of her head as if to say that our thoughts about Jimmy were in sync. I did not know what Jimmy had told her, or if it was even the same version that he had told me. But his blunt and unashamed approach with me made me certain that he would tell her the same story.

She took the cup from him and said, "I'll be back in a few to put you in the bed before those pills knock you out." She turned and strode confidently from the room, deliberately ignoring Jimmy's playful call, "Don't forget!"

"I will let you rest, but I want you to tell me one more thing."

"What you wanna know?"

"What do you think's going to happen with all this violence?" I asked.

Jimmy searched to gather an answer. "Man, this was the roughest year so far. I think it's going to continue and continue until there ain't nobody left, I guess. There's so many people out there that lost their boys or their cousins or somebody. They're going to want to get the person that did it, just like I would want to. So it ain't going to never end. I don't think it's going to ever end."

We stopped at this sobering place. Jimmy was starting to doze now, and his right eyelid intermittently sagged to the level of his left. The nurse reappeared and began to gather Jimmy for the slow and deliberate procedure of easing him back into the carefully made up bed. I thanked Jimmy and told him that I would be back to check on him.

"Do that," he said. "It's boring in here."

I left Jimmy's room and walked past the nurses' station painted with animated pumpkins dancing on thick legs and wearing shoes like the pilgrims wore. I took the stairs down to the basement and then trekked through the dank tunnels, where bland paint peeled off the porous walls. When I got to my office, I began the familiar routine of checking my microcassette recorder to be sure that it had captured our conversation. I moved the switch into the play position and was relieved to hear the oddly nasal sound of my own voice and the more pinched tone of Jimmy's. I removed the cassette and wrapped it carefully in plastic bubble wrap. I slid it first into a padded envelope and then into a FedEx mailer. I addressed the form to the transcriber and walked the envelope back downstairs to the drop box outside the door to my building.

Over the next few days, I stopped in to see Jimmy each day. He improved noticeably each time I saw him. On Wednesday, he was walking the hall with a physical therapist. On Thursday, I found him sitting in the chair feeding himself. We talked, but we did not return to the topic of how he got shot. He seemed content to talk about other topics, like his restlessness at being so confined.

"This place is so boring. They only have little kid video games here. They tell me I might be able to go home on the weekend. I can't wait," he told me. "I gotta get out of here and back to my brothers and sisters." His speech was clearer, though his face was still densely limp.

"Good for you," I said. I could not resist asking what he would do once the surgeons sent him back to his family in the projects. "Jimmy, how do you think this whole experience will change life for you in the future?"

He tilted his head to the side with slight annoyance. "I really don't know. I really can't say."

"Well, why do you think all this happened?" I knew I was pressing.

"Why do I think that I got shot? My idea is that somebody that didn't get along with me paid him to do that. That's my idea because he's a bitch, you know what I'm saying? He's scared of me, so I think someone paid the dude to do it. So, I know he really didn't want to do it, but if somebody threw a few thousand dollars in his face, he probably just took it and did it. That's the only thing I could think of."

"How are you going to try to avoid anything else happening to you?" I asked.

"Avoid it?" He huffed. "I really can't avoid it because Boston's a small area. I been thinking about moving away, but I got to get my stuff together first, you know? I just ain't going to get out of the hospital and move out of here."

"And what about your safety? How are you going to stay safe if you stay in town?"

"I ain't saying that I'm untouchable, but I'm saying I ain't scared to die. I've been shot six times, so I ain't going to be scared to go where I'm going to go. I just got to be more careful."

"More careful?"

"Yeah. And if I have to go someplace by myself, I got a burner. I could always take that."

"A burner?" I asked.

"Yeah, a nina," Jimmy answered.

"What's that?" I questioned, again trying to break the code.

"A nine . . . a nine millimeter." He said this with complete calm, like he was telling me his address or what size shirt he wore.

"When do you carry it?" I asked.

"Sometimes, like sometimes when my conscience tells me to or if I get a feeling that something might happen."

"Where did you get a gun?"

"This dude in the neighborhood. He smokes crack. I just asked him, and he bought it for me."

I felt more worried about this little man than I had at any point before. He was transforming in front of me—with every word, every phrase, punctuated with nonchalance—from an injured patient into a young black man who could reason his way into hurting someone. His physical scars were easy for me to see, but he hid his other scars well behind the terse indifference in his voice.

I was tempted to probe deeper into the gun and what he might do with it, but a different question jumped into my mind—and mouth. "Jimmy, tell me this. What do you think it would take for there to be peace?"

As I had come to expect, he did not hesitate a beat. "No guns for nobody except the police. And that would be odd because there's guns everywhere. Everywhere. Everybody and their mama got guns, so it ain't going to ever stop."

His answer surprised me. This was not at all what I expected him to say on the heels of his own gun story.

"How would you do that, get rid of the guns?"

"I couldn't even say. I don't think there's a way because there's a lot of crackheads out there that got them cards that can get guns. You know what I'm saying?"

"What do you mean?"

"Yeah, they got licenses to buy guns. They can just go in and order you a whole shipment of them joints, so it ain't going to stop."

I stood there, saying nothing, unable to make sense of Jimmy's answer. Jimmy had a gun, but he wanted only the police to have guns, and it was "crackheads" who stood in the way of this. This must simply have been his way to say that there was no hope. I wanted to delve deeper and to try to find some hope but again, Jimmy preempted me.

"The only way out of this is to be saved, you know what I'm saying? That's the only way."

It took me a moment to catch his meaning. If I had not myself grown up in the Ebenezer Missionary Baptist Church in Flushing, New York, I might have missed that Jimmy was referring to spiritual salvation.

"So, you believe in God," I said.

"Yeah. I can't say I'm with Him, but I know He's there. But I do believe there's a God."

"And how does that affect your life?"

"Oh, it don't affect me. I just hope that one day I can be with Him. But right now, there's a lot happening. I just can't do it overnight, you know what I'm saying? But there should be a time. I just can't say when."

"That's good," I told him. This was a small offer of hope, and I accepted it for what it was. I knew from what other young men have told me that watching their blood flow freely from their bodies can bring them face to face with God. And I hoped it was something Jimmy could hold on to. He came by this honestly, I could tell. Throughout our conversations, Jimmy referenced his grandmother, the matriarch of the family. I could tell from his tone that he respected her. And without knowing much, I guessed that she was the one who gave him a spiritual sense to hang on to. I hoped that he might find something in this to break free of the hold the streets had on him.

■ ■ ■

It was nearly five in the evening when I found, in my inbox, the brown manila envelope containing the transcript of my talk with Jimmy. It had been two weeks since I had sat and talked with him, and in that time some of the details had faded from my memory. This was often the case. And it was not entirely a bad thing. There were ideas that were easy to hear when a young man was telling his story. But these were not necessarily the most important ones. Other thoughts and words and stories took shape only once the words had been set down on paper.

I walked back to my office and pulled out the thick stack of white paper. The sharp smell of the transcriber's stale cigarette smoke coated the paper and clung to my hands. I sank into my swivel chair and spread the pages like leaves across the desk, where I could move between the parts of our back and forth.

The words took on a new sense of urgency after being transformed from sound to ink. I became enveloped in his story and its rhythm as it ran across the pages. All of it seemed new and fresh, and there were whole portions that seemed unfamiliar at first, almost as if the interview had been done by someone else. But as I read further, the words transported me back to the brightly colored room, and I began to hear Jimmy's voice echoing in my ears and my head as though I were still there with him.

Though all of it was important and most of it familiar, something that Jimmy had said leaped out again at me with an unusual ring of familiarity. I looked at the pages where I asked him about what it meant to be a sucker and why young guys wanted to have a rep. He said, "Just to be known. People don't like to be nobodies these days. They like to be somebody or try to be somebody."

I spent an hour or so hunched over these papers, coursing in and out of Jimmy's words, trying to connect to them and understand them better. Buried within was an inherent logic that seeped up through the street words that Jimmy spoke. I slid my finger back and forth over the pages, drawing invisible arrows from one idea to the next.

A complex logic began to appear to me. I grabbed a scrap of

paper and sketched out the steps in the logic that Jimmy laid out. The notes fell out like this:

- If you want to avoid being a sucker, you have to have a rep.
- If you want to have a rep, you have to earn it.
- You earn a rep by putting in work.
- In Jimmy's world, work means doing violence.
- Having a rep, even if you got it by violence, makes you known.
- When you are known, you are somebody.
- You could get a rep for doing good, but people might still come after you for disrespecting them in the past. Therefore violence is more effective.

The logic was simple, almost elegant, so coherent that I found it deeply disturbing. I had gotten used to talking about senseless violence. How could violence be anything but senseless? Hundreds of young people wounded, dozens of young black men dead. This suffering was hard for me to get my head around. At first it made no sense to me.

But Jimmy's argument, when I laid it out in front of me, told me that violence made sense to him. Violence worked in his world to accomplish something that all of us wanted—to be somebody—but that Jimmy could not find any other way to do. I flipped through past interviews in my mind and realized that I had seen fragments of the same argument in the dense commentaries that cushion the black males' injury narratives. But I didn't know how widespread this idea was. I knew that most of the young men I talked to could define the term *sucker* without even stopping to think about it. But whether they linked their very identities to the idea was not something I could have imagined.

There was another troubling implication here too. If I heard Jimmy right, he was implying this: if you face danger trying to get a rep by doing good, why not get a rep using something that may shield you from peril? Why not use violence to make your mark on the world?

■ ■ ■

Several months later, I was sitting in my office late one afternoon when Roy stopped by. Roy had made it a habit of popping by once or twice a week on his way home from his new job. Remarkably, a number of mentors and associates of the CLUB program had recognized how brilliant Roy was. As a result, Roy had landed an internship in the office of John Kerry, the U.S. senator from Massachusetts. This was a major leap forward for someone who only weeks earlier was confined to the stifling routine of a prison prerelease center.

As usual, Roy was wearing a suit. Today he sported a moss green, double-breasted, cotton and polyester Macy's special that was beginning to shine with age. He carried a small Adidas gym bag. Roy came into the office and stood near the door with his usual greeting: "So what's going on?"

"Just working," I said.

"This late?"

I laughed and looked at the desk clock, which showed 5:17 p.m. "This isn't really late," I told him. "Going to the gym?" I asked. Roy seemed not to understand, but then gripped his bag as if it had magically appeared in his hand.

"Oh, this? Nah. I just carry my hoodie in it," he answered referring to his black hooded sweatshirt.

"Your hoodie? What for?"

"Not a good idea to walk down my street like this," he said, sweeping his hand down across his suit and tie. "I'm not trying to stick out like that. So I cover it with the hoodie until I get out of the neighborhood. Then I take it off when I get downtown. That way nobody messes with me."

"Hmmmm," I said, for lack of a better word. "Is it that bad?"

"Yeah, man," he said, smiling as if the question understated the problem. He looked around for a place to set down his bag.

"Pull up a chair and check this out with me." I told him that I had recently spoken with a young man who had been shot in a gang-related battle. Then, without revealing anything about Jimmy himself, I read to Roy the brief section of the interview where Jimmy talked about being "known."

"Does that make sense to you?" I asked.

Roy leaned back in the swivel chair so it bounced on its springs. "Yeah," he said, never taking his eyes off me. "That makes perfect sense."

At this point, Roy began to drift into a tone of voice that I had become familiar with. His voice hardened and developed a sharper edge. His voice grew louder and would have sounded argumentative if I had not heard this tone many times before.

When I first heard him use this voice at one of the meetings of the mentoring program where he and I had met, the voice sounded bruising, almost chastising. But over time, I had come to understand this as his strident voice, a voice that carried a kind of passion masked by a muted disgust. He became like a teacher lecturing on some unpleasant and unseemly episode in modern history. It was as if Roy knew the answer so deeply and so personally that it pissed him off.

"It's like any kid growing up in the ghetto. You look around and what do you see? You don't see a lot of folks like yourself goin' off to work, 'cause even if they are there, you don't really see them. They leave their houses early in the morning, and you don't see them when they come home. And think about it, none of those folks interact with young dudes like this young brother, so it's almost like both crowds don't exist to each other, almost like walking past squirrels. We just exist on the planet together, but we ain't the same."

"So help me understand how that makes somebody violent or gets them shot. Just because those folks don't acknowledge you or interact with you, people get hurt or get violent?"

"Naw, but I can tell you this: when a person gets treated like he don't exist, that person feels like he's inadequate or you look down on him—or you think he ain't nothing compared to you."

"Well, where does the violence come in?" I asked.

"Simple. The logic in his head is this, 'You might be better than me, but I bet I can fuck you up. Who's the man now? I bet you'll respect me now.' "

Roy paused. "What does this kid look like?" Roy suddenly asked, in an apparent change of subject.

"Why do you ask?"

"I bet this kid isn't the kind of kid who's gonna be a basketball star. Or a lady's man, a player, right?" Roy said, answering his own question. "He probably ain't no great brainiac who's going to college. If he was any of those things, he would be doing that. He'd be about that kind of stuff. But he's not."

"I follow what you're saying," I said. "But let me push back a little, because I don't believe that's what made him a victim. Anybody can become a victim; I don't buy the logic that everybody that gets hurt brought it on themselves."

"I'm not saying that's what made him a victim, but it pushed him in that direction. That's why this kid's a gangster. In his mind, that's all he's got available to him. He wants to be known for something. Athletes are known for being athletes, players are known for being players, academics are known for academics. That's why they get a pass in the hood. You know what they are and you know what they're about.

"Think about it: those who can't be famous settle on being infamous. They say the same thing this kid says, 'At least I'm known, at least I ain't a nobody.' That's the thinking. They want to fit in somewhere.

"So if I'm this kid and I'm in the neighborhood and everybody around me is trying to act like they're 'all that,' and I ain't shit? Well I might just fuck them up or rob them to prove that 'I am somebody.' It's like, 'If you can't respect me, then fear me.' So if they don't acknowledge his humanity and he ain't allowed to exist among the respect community, then he'll be a part of the fear community, and fuck with their humanity. You get this?" Roy unexpectedly popped out of the chair and his face grew more severe.

"It's like you," he said. "You do this research. You write ar-

ticles. You want your colleagues to know you, to know the kind
of stuff you're doing, right?"

"Uh, yeah, I suppose," I said slowly, unclear where he was
going.

"And your colleagues are your community, right?"

"Yeah, I guess so . . ."

"Well, it's the same for him."

The comparison caught me off guard. I found Roy's implication, that Jimmy and I had the same motives, to be both
amusing and irritating. But I let it go without comment for the
moment.

Roy went on, hitting his stride now. "Just like athletes are a
community, church people are a community, dudes who play
the girls are a community. But some of us don't belong nowhere, and the streets are the last place for some of us to find a
community. Nobody wants to be a nobody. Nobody wants to
be without a community. Even homeless people have a community. We all want to belong somewhere or belong to somebody.

"Think about this, Doc: What would you be if you *weren't*
a doctor? Think about yourself right now, could you see yourself being satisfied with your existence if you flipped burgers
for a living?"

"I hear you, and I'm not sure I agree, but go on."

Roy was on fire now. Roy was a willing teacher but he also
rarely demurred from a challenge to argue. "You don't? Well
just think about it. This is your own little doctor world. All the
doctors are working, trying to stand out from the other doctors. There's probably some guys who just automatically stand
out because they make all the money or they're doin' brain surgery or something. Shit, y'all probably have your own version
of doctor competition or doctor cliques or gangs. You might
even have doctor haters that try to sabotage shit.

"Some people are just always gonna stand out. Some people
are going to hate that, too. But then there's a lot of other people
who are tryin' to get attention. Trying to make a reputation.

You do your work. You put it out there. You work hard. And you want somebody to notice it. Right?"

Roy didn't wait for my response.

"Of course you do," he said, answering for me.

Perhaps seeing the lines developing in my brow, Roy softened, but only to make his point. "Now you know it's not like I'm saying that you are like a gangster or something like that. You're trying to do good, save people's lives. And that is what you're a part of, I get that. But this kid wants somebody to know him too and be a part of something too.

"And just like if nobody noticed the work you do, you would end up a nobody? Think about who you would be then? Well, it's the same for him. There's lots of kids out there acting crazy just trying to get somebody to know who they are. I know, 'cause I was one of them. I did my dirt in the streets. And I suffered for it. But the more I think about what little dude is sayin', you know he's kinda right. Even now, I can walk through the projects, and people don't mess with me 'cause they know me. Even though I'm not still in the game, people know my track record, so they usually pick somebody else to test instead of me. A young kid in the neighborhood might be attracted to that, and they try to get close to me to get the same kind of respect, attention, or recognition that I get. He might even be willing to do dangerous things to impress me to get my attention. All kids do that."

"Say more," I prodded.

"There's lots of kids out there just like this kid. Believe it. Younger kids have tantrums to get attention, right? Well, danger gets you attention. That shit's been working forever."

In the moments that I had been listening intently to Roy, my momentary offense had passed. I found myself enveloped in Roy's reasoning, and my mind flicked back and forth between Jimmy's explanation and Roy's analysis. If Roy was right, the perspective seemed overwhelmingly gloomy. *If I can't be famous, I'll settle for being infamous.* There might be hundreds of young men out there raised by weakened, drug-addicted parents, dropouts from schools that couldn't hold them, disappointed by fathers who deserted them without stopping to explain their own scars. If these young men were numb from all the violence that they had seen and if they, like Jimmy, were unable to see a clear future, then the whole concept of violence in the inner city was beginning to make sense.

That it did make sense unsettled me. But with Roy's help I was starting to understand that there was something about violence and the retribution that spilled out into the streets in the neighborhoods that made sense. The other young men who had hinted at the same idea over the previous few months had seemed so enmeshed in the gang world that I had dismissed the ideas as gang ideas. At that point, I thought they were just telling me what young men in gangs thought. When Jimmy took me on a tour of the same logic in his mind, it became clearer to me that many young men shared this logic, especially since so many young patients knew just what they needed to do to avoid becoming a sucker.

Now with Roy standing in front of me laying it out by drawing parallels to my own life and career, I couldn't miss it any longer.

So I turned to Roy. "So what about you? What do you see in the future for you to keep you out of the streets?"

Roy bent his knees to slide back into the chair. He looked pensive and slightly concerned by the question.

"You know, I think about this a lot. And I can't say that I have it all figured out. I really don't know. I just hope doing right is gonna pay off someday. I ain't all churchy and shit, but I believe in God. So I just believe that being good has to pay off someday. At least it's supposed to. Right now, I'm going to work every day, looking for a better gig every day, but at the same time, I got kids, man, and I love 'em, so I gotta stay straight, and just have faith that being good will give me the answers I need.

"But in a lot of ways, I was doing better when I was doing bad than I am now that I'm doin' good. I make $400 a week in a good week. I used to make $400 a *sale* easy, on a usual day on the block. I had a lot more money when I was doing that. I also had a lot more to worry about, too."

"Like going back to jail?"

"Kind of, but not just going back to prison. Prison wasn't shit. I was known in prison before I got there."

"So what were you worried about? Getting caught? Or letting people down?"

"Honestly?"

"Yeah, if you don't mind."

"I was worried about the prayer."

"Explain."

"Everybody that gets locked up says the same prayer when the steel doors slam, 'God, if you get me out of this one, I swear I'll never . . .' prayer. Seriously, and everybody that gets shot says the same prayer too! But then as soon as you get back in order, you're back doing the same bullshit. So the last time I got locked up, I actually asked God to 'Give me what I deserve this time and not what I want, and not what the judge wants to give me,' because I'd said that prayer a million times and went back on my word. So in my heart I thought God was slapping me up. So this time, I didn't make the same prayer, and I promised myself that I would really try hard this time, and if being good didn't work, it wasn't meant to work, and I could at least say to God the next time that I really tried.

"So I would rather worry about how to pay for sneakers and school clothes and all the other stuff kids need than to worry about if I am gonna wind up in jail, lying to God again.

"I think it is better not to be able to give them all the stuff they need than to not be able to give them the love that they need. So it's tough, but if my honest attempts at being good didn't pay off, then yeah, I'd go all the way *back into the game.*"

"I get it," I told him, "and I appreciate it."

"You got it," Roy said. He bent to pick up his bag.

"You can put your hoodie on in here, if you want," I told him, pointing to the bag.

Roy laughed. "Nah, I'm cool. I don't need it until I get down closer to home."

Roy left, and I sat and thought about what he had taught me. I began to see some parallels between what Jimmy and Roy were telling me. Both Jimmy and Roy were talking about how they protected themselves in the streets. Even Roy's hoodie disguise spoke of the image he had to project to stay safe. Roy confirmed what Jimmy was arguing: being known kept their enemies at bay. Being respected was a form of self-defense.

But Jimmy was using violence for something even more fundamental—and Roy helped me see this fact. Jimmy was using violence to build an identity in the same way the rest of us use school and family and occupation. He was using the chaos and violence of the streets to be the only *somebody* that he believed he could be. It goes without saying, since Jimmy used violence to gain street credibility and become *somebody*, that the person who wounds or kills Jimmy will gain street cred. Thus the continuity of violence, havoc, and death in the streets of the inner cities.

Most of my colleagues believed that the problems these young men displayed were their own fault. They believed that these men simply made bad choices in the midst of a land of opportunity and that these bad choices got them in trouble. Some would admit that poverty played a role. A few would admit that discrimination was a part of the problem.

But I sat there and imagined myself standing in an auditorium filled with my colleagues, putting forth the idea that these young black men were using violence to construct a respected identity, just like everyone else does. I imagined that I would be laughed out of the room. There was about as much tolerance for the idea that violence had a logical explanation as there was for the idea that not all of these young men are criminals.

A seasoned trauma surgeon once pulled me aside when I suggested that a young man with a gunshot wound had not provoked the attack. He told me, "Any time one of these kids gets shot and either dies or is very sick, immediately he was the valedictorian of the high school, the best football player, the churchgoer—I mean, all these kids were the greatest kids. I mean, you'd think they were all accepted by Harvard. Bullshit! They know it's not true. They're a bunch of troublemakers. Some are lucky, some are less lucky, and some just get what they deserve."

And so, as disturbing as it was to me that Jimmy used violence and gangbanging to try to build an identity and to keep from vanishing into invisibility, the idea also gave me a sense of opportunity. For me, the belief that violence is senseless requires that we see these young men as purely bad, as savages who are injured and killed out of pure malice. I thought back to something my colleague Dr. Sandra Bloom, trauma psychiatrist, told me. Our tendency to demonize these young men requires that we classify them into one of two categories: sick or bad. Seeing them as sick implies that they bear no responsibility for their actions, that they are inherently defective, and that experts are needed to provide them with *treatment*. Seeing them as bad, on the other hand, implies that they bear all of the responsibility for the problem, that they are even more defective, and that what they need most is *punishment*.

But Dr. Bloom holds out a third possibility that changes the whole way we approach them. She suggests that we see them as *injured*. To do so does not relieve them of their responsibility; we merely recognize all the poverty and loss and violence and hopelessness that made them see the world as they do. It implies that all of us bear responsibility for understanding why they got injured and how to prevent it from happening again. Seeing them as injured also leads us to the conclusion that the remedy is *healing*.

Her insight offers hope that Jimmy, having recognized that being a tough guy had only brought him more pain, might come to believe that he could find another way to be somebody. His mother and father could not do this for him, since they too were searching for another path. I thought about my own journey. Had I not had such an example in my life in the person of my father, I might not have known that there was any future for me in medicine. More sobering was the thought that if I had grown up in the same place and conditions of trauma and violence that Jimmy had grown up in, I would likely see the same narrow horizon of possibilities that he saw.

4

JIMMY IN THE STREET

On a warm evening in late May, I pulled my car into the Mobil station on Blue Hill Avenue next to the Freedom Baptist Church. It was nearly 7 p.m., and the light was beginning to fade. As I was filling my tank with gas, I saw a teenager swoop by on a mountain bike and spin around by the air compressor. I squinted at the young man's wide face and neat cornrows. He looked familiar, but I couldn't tell for sure in the low light. He finished hastily putting air in the tires of his bike and hopped on. He rode back toward me, and I saw him more clearly.

"Hey man," I said, recognizing him as Jimmy.

A curious look came over his face for a second, but he suddenly recognized me.

"Hey . . . the doctor from City."

"That's right," I said. "Wow, you look completely better."

It had been almost a year since I last saw him. His hair was styled into pristine rows, and his crisp clothes looked as though they were being worn for the first time. His face bore none of the asymmetry that it had had in the hospital. When he spoke, his words were no longer slurred. Still, his voice was just as nasal when he talked.

"You doing okay?" I asked.

"Yep. All healed up."

"Great. No problems?"

"Nah, Doc, all that stuff blew over. It's squashed. I just stay away from those dudes."

He stayed on his bike as we chatted, looking around from time to time. He stood up on the bike pedals, lifted himself off the seat, and then settled back into the leather saddle. He seemed distracted and eager to finish this chat so he could ride off.

"Well, stop by and let us know how you are doing," I offered.

"Bet! I could give you my number," he said. I reached into my car and pulled out a scrap of paper and pen from the glove box. I took down his number. "That's my grandmother's," he said as he rolled away. "See you, Doc."

He pedaled away fast, looking pleased with his ability on the bike. He zigzagged across the pavement of the station like a skater cutting a figure on the ice and then swung out and away onto Blue Hill Avenue.

For months after that, I heard nothing from Jimmy, and I did not run into him on the streets. Still, I thought about him every time other young patients started to talk about making a rep and being known. Few of them have been able to explain it with the cool clarity that Jimmy had. And his voice played in my head each time the subject was raised.

Late one evening, I was sitting at my computer tapping out my own version of these ideas when I started thinking about Jimmy again. I pulled the small piece of paper from my wallet and looked at the number he gave me. I dialed it, and an elderly woman answered. "Hello, is Jimmy Parker there?"

"Who is this?" she asked with caution.

"This is Dr. Rich. I met Jimmy when he was here at the hospital after he got shot about a year ago. Is this Jimmy's grandmother?"

"Yes," she responded, still sounding suspicious.

"Well, I am just calling to see how he is doing."

She was quiet for a second.

"Well, he's in jail. Been there for a couple of months now."

"I'm sorry to hear that," I told her. "Do you mind telling me where he is, or his address? I would like to write him a letter."

"Hold on," she said sighing. She put the phone down and I could hear the sound of papers rustling. She gave me the address, to a facility labeled simply "MCI-Concord."

"Thank you," I said, hearing hesitancy and shame in her voice.

"Wait," she said. "You need his numbers too. 2-1-4-9-3-B. Put that on the letter and the envelope or else they won't give it to him."

"I'll do that," I told her. "Thank you again."

"Help him out. He needs it," she said. "All I can do now is pray for him." A sad resignation in her weak voice told me she had known that Jimmy would end up in jail but was powerless to stop it.

I hung up the phone and wondered just how he had ended up in jail, although the answer seemed obvious. He was wrapped up in the gang life. He called the person who shot him a "crime partner." But from the moment he lay in that hospital bed wincing in pain and drooling from his sagging lips, I hoped that he would find the moment of salvation he mentioned.

I sat down in front of my laptop and typed this short note.

Jimmy,

I don't know if you remember me, but I am the doctor who came to see you in the hospital a year ago when you got shot. I would like to hear about how you are doing. Please write me back if you have the chance. Hope to hear from you.

After a few weeks, a letter arrived in the mail bearing the stamp "Concord-MCI, Massachusetts Department of Corrections." Inside was a neatly handwritten letter.

Dr. Rich,

Thanks for your letter. I remember meeting you at City Hospital and I saw you that day at the gas station. I really appreciate that you wrote me a letter. I don't get too much mail here and so it was a nice surprise for a change.

I am only locked up here because of a mistaken identity. I have a lawyer who is working to help me appeal and get out. I hope I get out soon.

By the way, like I said, I do not get much mail, so if there is any way that you could send me a couple of dollars, I would really appreciate that. Up here, the only way that you can buy things like toothpaste and deodorant is to have a few dollars. Well, I'm messed up right now up here. I have 2 bars of soap left as of right now along with a dab of deodorant and toothpaste. And I wanted to ask you if you can send me a few dollars so that I can stock up on my cosmetics, whereas though I won't have to worry about them for at least another 5 or 6 months. I would totally appreciate that if you can do that for me, but if you can't squeeze it and you don't have it then I would understand, 'cause I know how it is out there. I know it's rough.

I hope that maybe even some day you might come up here to see me. I don't get many visitors. It's not too far from Boston, but I could tell you how to get here. So until I hear from you again, take care and be good out there. Peace Out!!

Jimmy

It felt good to hear from Jimmy. His letter was not dark but bright, upbeat. It was as though he were writing from camp—even the request for a few dollars had the ring of summer innocence. I was sad to think of him locked up in a state prison. But at the same time, I was relieved that he was safe from the menacing streets.

We exchanged letters several more times over the next 10 months. With each letter to him, I encouraged Jimmy to use the time productively, to work on his GED and learn as much as he could. Jimmy's letters reassured me that while he hated being there, he was using the time to read and study while also waiting for his lawyer's appeal to free him. Nearly every letter from Jimmy ended with two requests: one for a few dollars to get him toiletries and the other for me to visit him at Concord-MCI. The first request was relatively easy and could be satisfied with a $20 money order. The second request, to visit him in jail, gave me pause. Getting to Concord would take less than an hour. But I hated prisons. And my past experiences visiting inmates told me that I would spend most of the day navigating the stifling bureaucracy. Still, Jimmy had taught me so much, I knew that I could tolerate the annoying discomfort of that one day. I owed him that much, at least.

5

IN THE WRONG PLACE

Not long after I got that first letter from Jimmy, I went into the surgical ward to follow up on a young patient named Bryan. Several years before I met him, Bryan was shot in a drug deal that went bad; he wound up paralyzed from the waist down. He was confined to a wheelchair and every year or so would develop deep and difficult bedsores that would get infected with methicillin-resistant staph aureus (MRSA), a particularly tough bacterium to treat. The small conference room where the charts were kept was packed with interns, medical students, nursing students, physical therapists, and surgical attending physicians.

I pulled Bryan's chart off the rack and was leafing through the thick record when I heard loud voices coming in from the hallway. Most of the heads in the room bobbed up out of their books, and we all automatically listened to hear if the voices were those of catastrophe, such as a patient in cardiac arrest. But these voices bore the distinct edge of conflict. I heard first the young voice of a man, whose speech marked him as likely African American. I then heard the responding voice of a woman, perhaps a nurse. The exchange did not go on long, but

I could tell, even without being able to make out the words, that it was full of tension.

Within a minute, a stocky nurse in green scrubs and a blue smock appeared at the door. Her face was pink with agitation, and her brow was creased into a scowl. The surgeons and nurses at the tables looked up again as she entered.

"Animals!" she said loudly. "They're all animals!" She spoke to no one in particular. She simply propelled the words into the air, repeating herself as though she were waiting for the words to echo back to her. All of the people in the room simply returned their gazes to their books—the way subway riders look away when a mentally ill person is speaking to himself. The nurse was fuming. She walked over and snatched a chart from the rack. Then she turned toward a nurse sitting next to the rack and said again, "They're all animals."

Her final pronouncement was followed by a dense silence. No conversation, not even the rustling of movement. I said nothing either, even though my chest ached with anger. It was obvious to all of us that the patient she was talking about was a young black man. The words she was using, even if they were expressing some deep frustration, stung me, if only by association. I was the only black person in the room—and, obviously, a black man at that. I desperately wanted to speak out and to say something to challenge her, but I felt tremendous ambivalence. What she was saying was wrong, but it was not so different from the kinds of things that providers say when they enter a private space to vent their frustration. To her credit, she had not said this to the patient's face. At the same time, I took her words personally. I felt paralyzed to speak, in part because it would require so much explaining. What would I do? Chastise her by talking about issues of race and historical dehumanization of black men? Speak passionately about the slave times and Jim Crow and black protesters wearing placards around their necks declaring "I am a man"? I pictured the room full of people blinking at me as though it were now my turn to snap. Even a simple protest of "Don't call patients 'animals'" would sound self-righteous, would only call attention to me. This was the surgical ward, and I was merely passing through. So I simply stood and made my notes and stewed. I closed the chart and walked out, looking at no one and no one looking at me.

Halfway down the hall I ran into Cilorene Weekes-Cabey, whom we all knew as "Cil," the head nurse on the surgical floor and a friend. Cil was a tall and proud woman who had grown up in Monserrat in the British West Indies. Cil ruled the surgical floors with compassion and an iron hand. Nearly six feet tall, she wore her usual bright white pantsuit. Her smoothly permed brown hair fell off her shoulders and was streaked with an occasional wisp of gray. As the mother of two sons, she also had a special heart for the young men admitted to her floor. Like a mother, she comforted them and listened to them, but she also laid down the law when they became abusive or uncooperative.

I looked at her and she looked back at me. She could see the frustration in my face.

"Why that look?" she asked. "What's the matter?"

I vented to her about the scene that had just occurred, anxious to share my frustration with someone else. Was it just me? Was I being hypersensitive? She listened intently as I told her the story. I could see her mind working behind her eyes as she thought about her response.

She barely let me finish before declaring, "That's unacceptable. This is the same crap I deal with every day, and it's just got to stop. Now, you know some of these patients try to push our buttons. But we can't forget that we are professionals." Her words were sharp, and I knew that Cil was the kind of person who would just as soon put a misbehaving patient in his or her place as comfort the same patient during a painful moment. She was no pushover. Several times I had watched her read the riot act to a young guy who was manipulating a situation and creating chaos. But she also applied the same honesty to the nurses and physicians on the ward.

"I'm going to address this right now," she told me.

"That wasn't what I was trying to do," I told her, reversing my previous frustration. "I'm not trying to get anybody in trouble or get anybody fired. I just needed to vent."

"Nobody's getting anyone fired," she said. "They just need to learn. This is not tolerated."

She moved past me and started down the hall. She turned back. "I'm glad you told me. These are the kinds of things I need to hear."

I felt even worse than I had before. Now I felt not only my lack of courage to address the nurse's outburst myself but also the sinking feeling that engaging Cil would come back to haunt me or my patient in the future. I knew I would be back on these wards, either to see Bryan or to talk to other young patients who were injured. There was no way to avoid this nurse, and to be honest, I just didn't want to deal with it. It was not my job to tell my colleagues to refrain from calling patients "animals" or to urge them to stop thinking of them that way. But in a sense, that was exactly what I had done, albeit indirectly.

As I walked back to my office, I asked myself if the problem was theirs or mine. Hearing the nurse's voice of frustration aimed at the young black man evoked something in me. But the outrage I felt: was it about the treatment of this young man, or was it really about having my humanity impugned? In other words, if he was an animal, what then was I?

I thought back to the crusty trauma surgeon whose cynical view of these young men had stayed etched in my brain. I remembered another of his sarcastic pronouncements in response to my contention that not every victim fit the profile of a gang member: "Yeah, every last one of these guys was on his way to get a loaf of bread from the store for his mother when suddenly he got hit by a bullet. That's bullshit! I don't even ask them what happened, because they all lie." His was an extreme view, to be sure. But when I raised this topic with other colleagues who work with trauma victims as surgeons, there was a tendency to divide the victims into two camps: Patients were either completely innocent—struck by a random bullet—or else they were hardened drug dealers—there was no in-between. Often the assessment about which of these cut-and-dry categories fit a given patient was based not on the patient's own story but on what happened when the patient and doctor met after surgery, often the first time the doctor saw the patient awake or coherent. In the first few moments of this encounter, if the patient reacted calmly and gratefully or engaged in a conversation with the doctor, he was judged to be a likely innocent. If, on the other hand, he was reticent, avoided eye contact, grunted a monosyllabic answer, or complained about his care, he must have been doing something he should not have done. Why else, they reason, would he be so unpleasant? The patient's own account rarely came into play, because it was rarely heard.

But as I sat and thumbed through the transcribed stories of 25 or so young patients I talked to, I saw something more complex. I know that I spoke with these patients after a day or two lying in a hospital bed. In that time, they may have cooled off a bit, had a chance to think about how to make their way back into their neighborhoods. Some of these patients told me that they had been stabbed while someone tried to rob them. These patients talked about how others were jealous of the chains, coats, shoes, rings, and cars that they owned. For them, the chance of getting robbed was just a fact of life. A few others said that they had been caught by a random bullet sprayed out from a handgun in some unknown smoldering conflict on their block. For the most part, these stories were delivered with frankness and candor. To me they rang true, if only because the stories were rich with the simple irrelevant details that are often strikingly absent from purely invented tales.

On the other end of the spectrum were a few young men who freely admitted that they were involved in the gang life. These patients did not hold back on details either. They bared their arms to show me the gang tattoos and explained the intricacies of dealing drugs on the corner. They had their own rationale for what they did and sometimes justified it with tales of personal trauma. But they made no apology for it. Still their stories too bore the scars of living with poverty, growing up without a father, witnessing violence against their mothers and friends, and growing up in neighborhoods where getting and maintaining "respect" influenced every decision they made.

Between these two ends of the spectrum were the majority of the stories I heard. At the center of these stories was the idea of respect and the need to look and act tough to ward off those who might take advantage of you. Often the need to appear tough led to an *escalating argument*, the central story for a number of patients. Against the backdrop of respect, several patients found themselves in arguments that spiraled out of control, usually in the presence of alcohol or drugs. These arguments could erupt between friends or "associates" but whether about money or girls or some trivial slight, the stakes of losing were high, since losing could make the loser a "sucker." In this context, even simple disagreements spiraled to violence.

Other young men told me they were *objects of revenge*, meaning that they were targeted for revenge by someone who had perceived some sign of disrespect. This jumped out at me as the most common explanation for violent injury. One young man was targeted for revenge because someone had correctly figured out that he and his crew had shot at him the week before. Likewise, Jimmy believed that a former "crime partner" was out to get him.

But for most of the young patients in this category, their offense was nothing that they would expect to get shot for. The simple act of talking to the wrong girl at a club led to one young man being shot by her boyfriend in the parking lot. Other offenses were as small as bumping shoulders with someone. Even beating back a robber in public could result in that person seeking revenge for being humiliated in the street. That such small insults could lead to violent acts of retaliation made it seem absurd to assign blame to the victim. While from our own protected perches as health care providers it could be tempting to offer advice like "Don't go to clubs" or "Don't go out at night," these suggestions seemed to be asking these men to accept the brutality of being victimized.

A few other patients used the phrase "mistaken victim." For several of them, what this meant was: they knew who the intended victim was and were either with that person or standing nearby when the conflict erupted. Several did not know who the intended target was. They simply knew that no one had any reason to attack them. David, for example, whose story I relate in the next chapter, told me in bitter resignation to the violence that left him injured and took his cousin's life, "There was no reason to kill nobody. If they thought we were somebody else, they should have made sure first, you know? I feel like they didn't care. They just wanted to shoot somebody."

It struck me as I listened that the explanation rang more true when I considered that a lot of young men in the inner city tend to look alike because they dress alike. Just as Roy threw on a hoodie over his suit before leaving the projects, other young men dress to avoid sticking out in a crowd. This is part of the reason they seem to run together in the minds of the providers who encounter them in the chaos of a busy hospital. This ensemble of Timberland boots, hooded sweatshirt, and baggy jeans is the updated version of what sociologist Elijah Anderson terms "the urban uniform." The flip side of appearing inconspicuous is the possibility that an agitated assailant seeking revenge on some other young black man in jeans and a black hooded sweatshirt might end up harming the wrong person. But proving this theory to the police or family or doctors in the hospital can be difficult, because it involves proving a negative: there is no identifiable "beef" the young man can refer to since his entire argument is that there was no such "beef" to begin with. At the same time, given how even a very small perceived slight can lead to an act of revenge, some young patients must wonder if they unwittingly brought this upon themselves by flirting with the wrong woman or casting an angry glance at the wrong guy.

I flipped again through the pages on the desk to see if any other stories leaped out at me. The rest of the narratives included one young man stabbed by a girlfriend who learned that he was cheating on her, a young man who was stabbed while he was defending a family member in a fight, and a couple of patients whose cocaine addictions made them targets of the dealer they owed money.

I sat with some wonder as these types rolled around in my mind. There is no way for me to know, based on this small number of cases, just how common each of these scenarios really is. But one thing resonated with my own experience as a doctor, as I talked to these patients: There was far more texture and complexity to the violence that had occurred than we often acknowledged. And it followed that "guilty" and "innocent" were not the only potential categories into which we might place them.

Another question surfaced in my head, this time from my internal critic: How could I be so sure that these patients were telling the truth? I did not have a simple answer to this question. I could only answer with the gut sense that I have developed in my years as a physician interacting with patients whose health depends on trusting me enough to tell me the truth. I could reassure myself that these young men do not put themselves out there as "choirboys." Many acknowledge their past, if fleeting, involvement in drugs, petty crime, or gang life. That others acknowledged their own use of alcohol and marijuana led me to trust that there was, in this compilation of stories, the essence of truth. I also believed that having gotten some distance from the initial event, they had found time to struggle not only with their stories but also with the meaning of those stories. In that setting, in the hours that we sat together, their guards lowered and their defenses loosened. As the time progressed, their language relaxed, and they began to punctuate their stories with the more familiar language of the street. Simultaneously, their narratives blossomed with details so specific that they could only represent something real. But in the end, I had no better answer for the internal voice than to admit that I had no true test of the truth of their stories.

Finally, I rejected the question altogether. To me, it matters less whether the stories these young men told would have tallied with a video recording of the incident. In the end, the stories they told are their own truths, spoken from their perspectives and filled with their own understandings, not only of their injuries but also of the world in which all of us live. Their perception represents their reality. And so I accept the stories for what they are.

■ ■ ■

Several days later, I returned to the surgical ward to check on Bryan. As I expected, I came face to face with the same nurse who had launched into the tirade that had so troubled me. We approached one another contritely; she for her explosion of words and I for lacking the courage to confront her directly. She apologized for using the word *animal* to refer to a patient, but first she assured me that there was no tinge of racial thinking to her words. The patient had been uncooperative all shift long, she explained, and when he finally kicked over a full urinal—quite intentionally—while arguing with her about a dressing change, she just lost it. But it was not about his blackness, she told me. She was not a racist.

I listened to her, shifting uncomfortably. I let her know that I understood her frustration and explained how the words had struck me at that moment. She listened and nodded her own understanding. I could feel her sincerity, and I knew that she was not evil or overtly racist. I understood that all of us were marked by the trauma that swirled around us but that there was no safe place to air that trauma. Still, inside I wanted this conversation to end and for us to return to the customary denial that kept us moving with such dispatch throughout the day.

I thanked her for the conversation, and we turned away from each other, I to the rack of charts and she to the door. She offered the final word as she left the room. "You know, I love it here. I came to work here because I wanted to help. I wouldn't work anywhere else."

6

A STONE IN THE HEART

It was August, and as I walked through the hospital to my clinic, the afternoon was unseasonably dry, and the sun was brilliant. With weather like this, I expected many of my patients to skip their appointments. But it was not the case that day. By one o'clock, healthy-looking young men filled the waiting room. Most came in with the usual problems—acne, toothaches, rashes, knee pain—ailments that were easily diagnosed and treated.

A few patients had complaints that took more time. One young man spent several minutes telling me that he wanted to get "checked out" and "make sure everything is straight." I asked him directly: "What is bothering you that made you come in today?"

"I got burned," he told me—code for a penile "drip" or some other problem in his genital area that he believed he got from a sexual partner.

Another young man came in with a disability form for me to fill out. He had been unable to work since getting stabbed in the chest several months before. He was trying to get SSI—Supplemental Security Income, as federal disability payments are called officially—but he had already been turned down once. The form was long and detailed. It took me 15 minutes or so to complete it hastily, and this put me behind schedule.

In the midst of clinic, I felt my cell phone buzz on my hip, but I ignored it. By 4 o'clock, there was a lull, and I used this moment of calm to check my voicemail. I found only one message, a garbled one from Michael Collins, director of the summer jobs program at the local antipoverty agency. I could only make out part of the message, but what I could hear grabbed my attention: "One of my kids got shot last night." He indicated that the young man had been brought here, to City Hospital. I called over to the surgical floor in the hospital. The clerk told me that she could find only one new patient there with a gunshot wound.

"When did he come in?" I asked.

"Last night," she answered. "He might go home later today."

"What's his name?" I asked.

"David Simpson. He's in room 4205."

I assumed this was the young man Michael told me about, and I took his location as a good sign. Serious trauma patients went to the intensive care unit. Patients with minor gunshot wounds, those in which the bullet only passed through an arm or a leg but did not hit any major nerves or blood vessels, were often discharged the same day or the next. Physically, these patients were fine, but they were the ones I worried about the most. They didn't get the precious days of respite from the streets that helped to clear their heads and soothe their anger. Instead, still traumatized from getting shot, they were pushed out into the same neighborhoods where the conflicts that had led to violence were still smoldering. The odds were high that these traumatized patients would end up back in the hospital if they got caught up in retaliation.

On my way back from clinic, I climbed the stairs to the fourth floor of the inpatient building and walked down the quiet halls to David's room. It was after 5 p.m., and nearly all the laboratory and radiology services were closed. Patients were no longer being whisked off to MRIs and CT scans. Elective surgical cases were finished, and the operating rooms lay dormant, awaiting the next emergency.

Those patients who could eat were being served bland dinners of baked chicken, scoops of instant mashed potatoes, stubs of frozen green beans, and the ubiquitous green Jell-O. Many were being attended to by their families, who appeared after long days at work. They brought small, steaming containers of peas and rice, mashed sweet potatoes, or chicken and rice soup for ailing aunts or mothers. The voices that drifted from behind the drawn blue curtains revealed the sounds of comfort and laughter—but conflict and worry as well.

When I got to David's room, I found him lying beneath a white sheet with his arms folded behind his head. His eyes were locked on the television, which was thumping out a hip-hop music video.

"I'm Dr. Rich. Mike Collins is a friend of mine. He told me you were here." At the sound of his friend's name, David lit up.

"Mike? You know Mike? He's cool. I love him." David was upbeat, almost jovial, the opposite of what I expected, given what he had been through.

I asked about his wound. "It's hardly anything," he told me, lifting the sheet and pulling back the faded blue hospital gown to reveal a small gauze dressing on the left side of his belly. "The bullet just went in and out."

"That's a good thing," I said. "You're lucky. After you're better, can I talk to you a little bit more about what happened?"

"Sure. Anytime. I am going home tomorrow," he told me. "Michael has my number. I see him all the time at work." He turned his attention back to the blaring television.

I left, glad that he was doing all right. As soon as I got back to my office, I called Michael.

"'All right'? Didn't he tell you about his cousin?" he asked me.

"No. What about him?"

"His cousin got shot too, and he died at another hospital. You didn't get my message?"

"No, not all of it. Does David know this?" I asked.

"Of course he knows. He was there."

■ ■ ■

It was several weeks before I was able to reach David. By this time, he and his family were past the difficult days of burying his cousin. His gunshot wound was almost healed. He invited me to come and talk to him at his place in Roxbury. The day we chose was humid, and thick clouds hovered over the city. I was halfway to his house when it began to rain.

I parked in front of the building where he lived. The rain seemed to come down harder just as I was getting out of my car. I grabbed my briefcase from the back seat and jogged toward the drab brownstone building. It was pouring, and it did me no good to run. By the time I got to the door, I was soaked.

The building had a security system, but fortunately a workman was repairing the door. I stepped over him out of the rain and into the small lobby. He was an older black man in blue coveralls with a cigarette hanging from his lips. He barely looked up at me. "I'm just going to 15C," I told him. He continued to turn his screwdriver against the bolt in the door hinge. He raised his other hand to point vaguely down the hallway.

"Straight back," he told me.

The air in the dark hallway was moist and heavy with the faint smell of cooked onions. I walked halfway down the hall and found David standing at the door to meet me. He was taller than me, by about eight inches. His head was wrapped in a black wave cap, the kind that drapes down the back of one's neck. He was dressed in denim shorts and an orange and blue New York Knicks basketball jersey. He had blue flip-flops on his feet. His right arm bore an indigo and red tattoo that read "Antoine." His face was somber. He reached out to shake my hand. "I was listening for you. You're right on time."

He invited me into the sparsely furnished apartment. It held only an olive green couch, a wooden coffee table, a television, and a small stereo system. The large screen television was on, but the sound was muted. Images of bejeweled rappers and women in skimpy bikinis bounced on the screen.

"How long have you lived here?" I asked him.

"I don't," he told me. "This girl I know? Well, this is her place. I just come over here 'cause we talk. We just be kickin' it, watchin' movies. Whenever I start feelin' bad, I just come over here, and we just start kickin' it." He stopped for a moment and motioned me to sit down on the velour couch.

"See? I can't really kick it with my girl, because she's always like 'Tell me you love me,' shit like that. I can't really kick it with her like that. So I come over here and we be kickin' it about movies. We kick it about other people. We laugh. I laugh, when I don't want to think of . . . when I'm feelin' bad, I start laughin'. I try not to take it serious."

David sat down on the other end of the sofa and rubbed the furry green fabric back and forth with his hand. He looked straight at me with empty brown eyes, waiting for me to ask him what happened on that day several months ago when he was shot. When he began to talk, his voice was deep and blunt. His tone was matter of fact, almost annoyed, like he was weary of telling this story.

"All right. I was in an incident where me and my cousin had went to a housing development, Green Street Housing Development, and I wind up getting shot, and my cousin wind up getting killed." He paused for a moment, searching the floor with his eyes. "And, there is nowhere to go from there with that one."

David looked up at me as if that was all there was to say. I waited several seconds, seeing if he wanted to go on. But he simply looked at me, glancing away for a moment at the pouring rain outside the open window behind him and then back again at me.

"Can you just tell me a little bit more about what that day was like?" I coaxed.

David shifted his feet and slid them in and out of his flip-flops.

"All right," he consented. "Antoine had came and picked me up from my house, and we was on our way to our godmother's house. I was goin' to wash clothes, and he was goin' to just pick me up. Then we wound up leavin' the house, 'cause I had to go get some change. We wound up goin' to Stop & Shop to get some change. And then we wound up hookin' up with one of our friends to go see some girls over in the projects. As soon as we got there, we wound up gettin' shot."

He paused again and looked at me.

"That's really about as much as I really want to say about that."

"Can you say anything about what happened after you got shot?"

"Well, I wasn't really thinkin' too much when I was gettin' shot. But afterwards, when I got out the car, I seen my cousin layin' on the ground. I guess he must have got out the car at some point in time and ran. But I never seen it happen.

"Then, when I seen him on the ground, even though I was shot too, I had to run to him to see if Antoine was all right. When I ran to him, I noticed that this liquid was comin' from his pants. So, it was really tense. I can't really describe it, how it felt. But it was very unpleasant. It was a very unpleasant feeling.

"And then, they rolled him over. When they rolled him over, I seen his eyes. His eyes was lookin' straight up. Looked all glassy. Right then, I was hopin' that he'd be all right.

"And then, the police officers, they was all badgering me. They were talkin' about 'You know, tell us who did it right now. You know who did it.' They was all yellin' at me, I was on the stretcher, and they was askin' me questions I couldn't answer. So it was very hard. I was mad, but then again, it was just difficult. It was just a difficult time until I got to the hospital.

"And when I got to the hospital, and they started workin' on me, the only thing I was thinking about was my cousin, seein' how he was doin'. Then a couple of hours went by and then my mother came in, my mother and my father. Then my sisters and brother came in. They told me Antoine passed away. And I just started to cry."

He paused. His pain was not apparent in his voice or on his face or in his eyes. But I felt a wave of emotion, and my eyes filled for a moment, but I blinked the tears back. I paused to let him finish.

"Then they took me up to the hospital room. And it was all over the news. And then, the doctor, the police detectives came in. They was askin' a whole bunch of questions. The newspaper was callin' me up in the room and everything. I was gettin' a lot of attention that I didn't really want. That's as far as that went right there."

David hesitated and stretched his legs out in front of him. He stayed like this for a moment and then jumped up and walked into the next room. He came back with a framed photo and held it up in front of me.

"This is Antoine and me when we was together in Greensboro, kickin' it at the North Carolina A&T homecoming."

The picture showed David and Antoine in front of packed stands at a football game. They were leaning on each other, and David had his arm draped over his cousin's shoulder. Each was holding a clenched fist against his chest. They both wore large grins on their faces, and their eyes reflected red from the camera flash. Like mirror images, each man's neck was hung with a gold chain. Their feet sported bright white Nikes.

"Antoine and me used to be like together every day. You know how it is. You grow up together, y'all become best friends. Some friends, they grow up, and they just grow apart. We grew up, and we grew together.

"Even when Antoine went to jail for like a year and a half. Even when he was in jail, we was writin' on the regular. Even though I didn't really go up to visit him, we stayed in contact on a regular basis. And then when he got out of jail, we was together every day. Every day.

"But then I wind up goin' to jail as soon as he got out. Matter o' fact, like a few months after he got outta jail, I went to jail for like four months. But we were still communicatin'. He was writin' me, I was writin' him. I was showin' him love. He was showin' me love. Then when I got outta jail, we was together every day. Like, even on the day it happened. We was together that day.

"We was like real close. It got to the point where I'd know what he was thinkin', and he knew what I was thinkin'. That's how close we became. And then this whole incident happened."

David drew another long breath and licked his dry lips. "My cousin Eric, Antoine's brother, was the last person who was with him before he died. He said Antoine told him to go check on me. That's the part that hurt the most. Yeah. His last word was like, 'Go see if David is all right.'

"So, you know what I'm sayin'? I was up here thinkin' about him. At the same time, he was up there, wonderin' about me. That really affected me. That really hurt. I don't think nobody can actually feel what I went through. Can't nobody really understand it."

David told me that the next time that he saw Antoine, it was through a plate glass window at the city morgue. David and his cousin Eric stood in a small room, and a curtain was pulled back to reveal Antoine's body. Until David saw the lifeless body of his cousin, he had continued to hope that somehow there had been a mistake; this was some other unfortunate black man. He fantasized that maybe Antoine was still gripping onto life in another bed in another hospital, mistaken for the one lying behind the curtain. But when the curtain was pulled back, his worst fear was made real.

"When we went to the morgue to identify Antoine's body, we seen that his mouth was open. And when they showed him to me behind the glass window, I just got real mad, because I seen his mouth open. Again, a whole lot of questions came to my mind. Like, 'Why is his mouth open?'

"So later, I went to my mother, because every time I had somethin' to ask, she had all the answers. I was like, 'You remember when we went to see Antoine, right? His mouth was open. It was like just dropped.'

"So she started gettin' spiritual on me. She started tellin' me when somebody's mouth is open, that's where they spirit leaves out of. And I believed that. Because it was just dropped open. It was a stunner. That just got me.

"I used to have religion. Like, I used to believe like there was a God, life after death. I still believe there's a God, but as far as life after death? I'm still like in the middle. I don't even know about that now.

"When I was in the hospital, I wanted to know why I was still here. Because the way that incident was, I shouldn't have even been here either. But for some reason I survived it. But I didn't feel that I was supposed to.

"And then I just started havin' all these dreams and everything. It just started messin' me up. So I tried to not think about it so much. But every now and then, a memory will come back, and I can feel it.

"When I go to sleep now, he's in a lot of my dreams. I don't be dreaming most of the time. But when I dream, he's in 'em.

"And sometimes, I can actually see the grave. It's like I'm inside his head. I can feel how it is to be in a grave. I don't like that feeling. Every now and then, I can actually see myself gettin' put in the ground."

David breathed in deeply. I said nothing. I couldn't come up with any words that would console him, and I didn't try. So I simply sat and looked at the same small place on the carpet where David had fixed his eyes. At first, it seemed that he might cry, but he just stared as if he had been transported somewhere else or was searching the ground for something he lost.

He looked up at me calmly. There was something about how David came across that took me a while to figure out. There was a disturbing disconnect between the painful moments he was describing and the ordinary look on his face and calm sound of his voice. The seeming inconsistency made him seem as though he didn't care about what had happened or that perhaps he was making it up. I knew that neither of these was true. Rather, his numbness was a result of the shock of losing his cousin.

"So me and Antoine's brother Eric are gettin' real close now. His birthday was last week, so we went out. And after we came back from goin' out, it was just me and Eric in the car. And he just started cryin'. He said 'David, they killed my brother.' And I had to hold him, like, 'It's gonna be all right.' But he broke down, 'cause he felt his brother should have been there wit' him on his birthday, 'cause his brother was *always* there wit' him on his birthday. And he just broke down. And the only thing I could say was 'Don't worry about it.'"

David flopped back in the chair and sucked his teeth with annoyance. "Now, the dudes who did it, there's mad hate towards them. I hate 'em. I can't say it any other way, you know what I'm sayin'? I'm not gonna risk puttin' myself in jail because of this and mess up the rest of my life the way they already messed it up. But I really don't like 'em. Matter of fact, I can't stand them boys.

"Now, I'm hopin' that what goes around comes back around. I can't wait for it to come back round to them, 'cause they took someone who was really, really special away from a lot of people . . . for nothin'. There was no reason to kill nobody. There was no reason to kill."

David jumped up from his chair now and paced to the door before turning back toward me. "If they thought we were somebody else, they should have made sure first. You know?"

He posed the question rhetorically, and there was nothing I could say. David had ventured into the seemingly illogical argument that the shooting would have been all right if the shooters had killed the people they intended to kill. I knew he meant something different, but I could tell that he had been trying to make sense of losing Antoine in any way he could.

David dropped his hands at my silence and slid slowly back to his place on the couch.

"I feel like they didn't care. They just wanted to shoot somebody. That's how I feel about it."

I asked David how all of this had changed him. David shuddered and shook his head. "A couple of minutes changed everything for me. A couple of minutes changed my whole outlook on everything. This thing really fucked me up. It really changed me."

"How?" I asked.

"Some things I used to be nervous about, scared about? I'm not scared of it no more. I feel that I've already been through the worst. Like a lot of things that made me scared or made me nervous, they don't scare me no more. They don't affect me.

"Used to be, if a whole bunch of dudes kept on lookin' at me, I used to feel nervous. Like if someone kept on like giving me mean looks? I used to get nervous. But that don't happen no more. It just don't happen. It's like some of the feelin' is just gone.

"If they look at me mean now, I look at 'em right back. Like, 'What?'

"It's like they just took some emotions that I used to have. That nervous feeling, that scared feeling? It's gone."

"Is that a good thing or a bad thing?" I asked naively.

"I think that's a bad thing," David said clearly. "I think I lost emotions over this whole thing. I lost emotions. I think my heart got a little stone in it now.

"And like I told you, my girlfriend gets mad at me now. She thinks I don't care no more, because I don't show it. And it's hurtin' her. But I've been tryin'.

"I can feel where she's comin' from, but I speak wit' my head now. I don't speak it right here, in my heart?" David thumped his finger on the orange number on his jersey for emphasis.

"I know she's good for me, but since this whole thing happened, I don't give a damn what she do. And this is somebody

I used to care about a lot. Now, I be like, 'I don't give a fuck. If you want to be with somebody else, go ahead.'

"I lost a lot of emotion over this. And I don't even know if it's gonna come back. I'm hopin' that it do, but you know what I'm saying? I care, but if it happens, it happens. If she leaves, she leaves. Life goes on. So I can't really call it."

David held the framed photo of Antoine up again for a moment before laying it down gently on the sofa. He leaned back and folded his arms across his chest.

"And now my performance at work is startin' to slip a little. I supervise kids in the summer youth work program, and this is the busiest time of the year. And I can feel it. I know it. I think I went back to work too early, because I went back to work like the followin' week. That was too early, 'cause now my work is startin' to really stress me.

"I took today off, because I was feelin' real stressed. My bosses have been tryin' to help me. They suggest I should talk to someone, 'cause I always talk to my boss, Michael. I love him because he gave me a chance when I got out of jail. Because when you get out of jail, you ain't supposed to get no job. Or at least it takes a while for you to get a job. He gave me a job right off the bat. He came up to see me in jail and everything. So I was like, the best thing I can do to repay him is just change everything."

■ ■ ■

By the time I walked out of the building, the rain had stopped and the sky was beginning to clear. I stepped around the puddles and back to my green Acura Integra. I drove down American Legion Highway splashing through the large pools along the lush edge of Franklin Park.

David's words echoed in my head. *I think my heart got a little stone in it now.* There was a medical diagnosis here, and I was poised to use the term post-traumatic stress disorder or PTSD. But sorting him into this sterile medical container did nothing for my understanding. In fact, I felt that to assign a diagnosis so casually was to turn my back on the young man, the living, breathing human being with whom I had just shared several hours.

I do know that David saw and dreamed about his cousin on the ground, in the morgue. He felt himself being lowered into the grave. He lived his life suspended between the reality of Antoine's death and his own emotions—the equivalent of the lay term *shock*. He was alternately sad and angry, like other young men who have been shot.

But there was something about David that was different. Most of my patients who had been through David's kind of trauma usually also showed "hypervigilance," the heightened sense of arousal that these young men often called "jumpiness." To these patients, every shadow and any loud noise could make them startle. When they passed other young men wearing the typical clothes of the inner city, they had to contain the overwhelming dread that carried them back to the attack. For them, this reexperiencing of the trauma became a real problem. They were pinned at home by their fear. They could not get on the T (Boston's subway) or ride the bus to a doctor's appointment or a job interview. When they did venture into public, they were twitchy, constantly scanning the faces around them. Their jumpiness made them look suspicious, as though they were about to rob the riders of the MBTA bus or snatch the purse of the next passerby. I have watched these young men sitting in the waiting room at the clinic, and they were often steeped in a wariness and fear that emanated from them like perspiration.

But David did not give off the vibrations of fear and anxiety. On the contrary, he was completely numb. I could not easily recall talking to any patient who had so completely lost his ability to feel. This symptom truly worried me.

David was worried too. He knew that his inability to feel love for his girlfriend could destroy their relationship. Without her, he was cut off from her love and the comfort she tried to bring. But he could not find words to explain to her why he was so unresponsive. He could only escape into the apartment of a woman who made him laugh.

But it was the loss of any sensation of fear that could threaten his life. I could imagine David with his new heart of stone, making his way through the streets of Roxbury, chasing down rumors that might lead him to his cousin's killers. If he believed such rumors to be true (although much of this street talk is not), would he confront the supposed shooters? Would he try and avenge Antoine's death? Would he act on bad information and hurt someone who had nothing to do with the shooting?

I couldn't answer these questions, since I knew little about this aspect of violence. For me, as for most of my colleagues in medicine, violence had clear, well-defined boundaries. For us, David's story began when he rolled through the doors of the emergency room and into the trauma bay. It continued into the operating room, then into his hospital bed onto the fourth floor. The story receded after a few days, when his wound started to heal and he could be discharged back home. He might come back in a couple of weeks to have the wound checked and the sutures removed. He might not. But either way, the story of violence—David's story—ended there.

We missed the moments of terror and pain that came before his arrival at the hospital. These moments seemed irrelevant to the critical tasks of repairing his penetrated body, replenishing his lost blood, restoring his blood pressure, checking his wounds, ordering more pain medications, shepherding the authorized visitors in and out of his room, consulting with the discharge planners, writing the prescriptions and the discharge orders, and caring for the many other patients who needed care and attention.

Likewise, on the other end of his trauma, we seldom saw the deeper scars that remained when he left the hospital physically healed but emotionally crippled. His life was now derailed. He was disconnected from his girlfriend because he could no longer feel love. He was angry and confrontational because he was newly numb to fear even when he came face to face with other young men who knew never to back down from a fight. Yet these were not our immediate concerns.

I was taught that these moments were outside the bounds of my role as a doctor. David was, after all, alive. He had recovered, survived—all of the good outcomes that he can expect from medical care. This was something he should be grateful for, whether he was or not.

And soon another injured young man would roll through the emergency department doors. We moved on. But the emotional scars that might fester in David's mind and drive him to drugs or violence were essentially invisible to us.

I had seen shadows of these scars in my young patients who came to the clinic with vague complaints and pains. They seemed anxious, off-balance, and unable to right themselves. They looked lost. They smoked marijuana rolled up into fat Phillies Blunt or Garcia Vega cigars bought at an inner-city convenience store. They choked down three or four a day, sometimes alone, sometimes with friends, trying to smoke away their unspoken pain.

Now, having sat with David and heard the dull voice and watched the empty fearless gaze, I could begin to connect the dots. These changes inside him were not just the result of grief and anger and bitterness and regret, even though doubtless these feelings were there. What David told me is that he was fundamentally different in some way that he could not explain. And the change left him unable to love the people he used to love and unable to fear the people he needed to fear.

■ ■ ■

I turned down Blue Hill Avenue and hung a left onto Warren Street. By this time, the rain had stopped, and the late afternoon sun had burned through the remaining clouds. Men and women, mostly black and Latino, had resumed their shopping and commuting through the bus station in Dudley Square. Cars pulled out of the parking lot of the Caribbean grocery store on Dudley Street and merged with the traffic inching toward Melnea Cass Boulevard. I navigated slowly through the mass of cars and people. An elderly Latina woman struggled quickly across the street toward the No. 42 bus. Coarse brown yams and leafy greens peeked over the edge of her heavy bag. I let her pass while three or four cars shot out in front of me. One of them screeched to a stop just a foot or two in front of the woman, and she continued on, undaunted, to the waiting bus.

I crept across the gridlocked intersection, and Washington Street finally cleared out along Ramsey Park. Over in the playground a collection of photos, teddy bears, botanical candles, and half-filled bottles of Hennessy surrounded a small elm tree by the basketball courts. This elaborate shrine, one of many that had sprung up of late, marked the spot where a young man had been gunned down some weeks earlier. Illuminated now by the sun, it looked surprisingly undamaged by the rain. Nearby, three young boys were shooting baskets, dribbling between the evaporating puddles.

I turned onto Northampton Street and pulled into the gray concrete parking garage. I usually cut through the hospital on my way back to the office but I chose instead to walk in the bright sun. I strolled to the corner and turned onto Albany Street. Just across Massachusetts Avenue, I passed the entrance to the emergency department, where an EMT was pulling a gurney out of the back of an ambulance. A thin, elderly black woman sat bolt upright, tightly gripping the rails of the stretcher. Her distressed eyes were open wide. Her nose and mouth were hidden behind the befogged oxygen mask pressed tightly to her face. As she struggled to breathe, her chest rose and fell, and the mask flashed first white, then clear, then white again. The EMT spun the stretcher around, and they disappeared through the automatic doors of the ED.

I kept walking past the main hospital toward the office of the chief medical examiner for Massachusetts. This new red brick building was home to the city morgue. Its clean structure was the image that I saw when I looked out of the window in my office. Although I saw this building every day, I was barely conscious of it. Considering that it held the bodies of so many young people tragically killed by violence or accidents, the place was surprisingly quiet. Cars and vans pulled in and out of the parking lot throughout the day, but they did not sound their sirens or race out and in. Whatever human contents they carried were unloaded unceremoniously behind the building and taken into the autopsy rooms. This routine of death was just that—routine.

Normally, I didn't think much about what happened there. But today, my mind floated back to David and his cousin peering through the glass at Antoine's body. Scenes like this took place each day. This quiet building contained not only the remains of real people whose lives had ended in tragedy. It contained the wailing and anguish and spiritual confusion of the families summoned there to identify a brother or cousin or son. They quietly came and went in the shadow of the building that held my office.

■ ■ ■

Back in my cluttered office, I took a moment to gather myself. Medical tomes and public health journals crowded the bland grey aluminum shelves. All around me sat volumes about violence. On the floor under my computer table, stacks of journal articles lay in the same spot they had occupied for months, silently pleading to be filed.

These books and papers had some value. There were books that spoke the facts and figures about violence. They counted the dead bodies of black men and boys killed in rage or drunken stupor by other black men or boys. Government reports revealed how large the problem of violence is in cities across the United States. A report from the Bureau of Justice Statistics dispassionately enumerated the terrifying data. Black males 18 to 24 years old had the highest homicide victimization rates. Black males 18 to 24 years old had the highest homicide offending rates. Young black males were disproportionately involved in homicide, both as victims and offenders, relative to their share of the population. The cities that consistently led U.S. rankings—places like Camden, New Jersey; New Orleans, Louisiana; Gary, Indiana; Richmond, Virginia; Philadelphia, Pennsylvania; Baltimore, Maryland; Detroit, Michigan; and Compton, California—all happened to be places where African American people predominated.

These statistics did not move me anymore. I had grown too used to the count of dead bodies. To me these numbers rang like the NBC evening news of my childhood that every night announced the number of war casualties in Vietnam. At first the news was shocking, then it became a distraction. Finally it blended into the background, a nuisance, like a toilet that continues to run after the most recent flush.

Beyond these numbers, the books around me barely spoke to David's pain. For the most part, these books about violence ignored the psychological scars of trauma. There was little or nothing there about flashbacks and nightmares. The journal articles about trauma largely ignored young black men, leaving us to extrapolate findings from studies of combat veterans and victims of sexual assault. Even the studies of young black men seemed to forget those who survive, instead focusing only on the dead.

One book, *Creating Sanctuary*, written by my colleague Dr. Sandra Bloom, took me beyond the hopeless numbers and blind theories about young black men and violence. Dr. Bloom is a brilliant psychiatrist who has devoted her life to studying trauma and taking care of traumatized people. She had recently become a valued friend and teacher.

Dr. Bloom made this complicated subject elegantly plain to me. She explained it this way: Think of the traumatized mind the way you would think about a broken leg. If a man has an accident and breaks his right leg, then that leg is put in a cast, and he cannot use it. Since it is immobilized, it begins to wither or atrophy. It loses its strength. Without the use of his right leg, he must shift his weight to his left leg. Because the right leg is unavailable, the left leg inevitably gets stronger as it assumes the work of the right.

Applied to trauma, she writes:

> Like the leg in the cast, the emotions that are bound up and im-
> mobilized are unavailable for normal use, thus significantly re-
> stricting the range of emotional depth and breadth. When a leg is
> broken, muscles in the other leg often become hypertrophied or
> enlarged, throwing the usually well-balanced system out of align-
> ment. With broken emotions, a similar experience occurs because
> other emotions fill in for the dissociated feelings.

Her words described David perfectly. The mixture of fear and love that was present at the time of the trauma—fear that he would die, his intense love for his cousin—were "broken" by violence. His ability to love was broken when he saw Antoine on the ground, dying. Now this love was unavailable for him to connect with his girlfriend, since it would transport him back to the intense pain of that moment. Instead, he felt nothing.

Likewise, whenever David used to feel fear, as in times of danger, he instead felt something else. Sometimes he felt anger; sometimes he felt the horrible weight of numbness. But the bottom line was that he felt anything other than fear. He was protected because the painful emotion was "in a cast."

Dr. Bloom's explanation helped me to understand not only David's pain but the seemingly peculiar responses of many of the young men I saw in the hospital as well. But I feared for David even more. If these emotions did not heal, someday his anger could rise up in place of his fear. What if he then came face to face with someone who wanted to harm him or take his life?

■ ■ ■

I walked down the street toward Baron's house in the Cod-man Square section of Dorchester. Baron and I met two months earlier, when he came to the hospital with several deep stab wounds to his abdomen. The 19-year-old and his former friend had gotten into a dispute over a girl, and in a spontaneous street corner brawl, they stabbed each other. Both were transported to City Hospital, and each declined to tell the police or providers who had stabbed him. Consequently, unbeknownst to the doctors and nurses in the hospital, the two young men were admitted to the same floor in the hospital. Both were so badly injured that no conflicts erupted in the hospital, but both required more than a week to recover from surgery to repair torn intestines. Once they were able to eat and walk and withstand the pain of healing, they returned to their classic homes in the turbulent neighborhoods where their families lived and toiled and tried to raise their children.

Baron returned to his family home on Talbot Avenue. The house belonged to his uncle, who had cared for Baron since he was six months old. I remembered Baron telling me the first time we met, "I have no mother or father."

It was a grand house, beige with chestnut accents. But like most of the houses on this street, there were signs of aging and decay. The paint was peeling. A gutter pipe swung loose from the roofline. A shutter lay on the ground under the window where it had once been attached.

This century-old, wood-frame, two-family house was typical of the houses on this street and in this section of Dorchester. They were originally built for Irish working-class people, new immigrants to America in the early 1900s. Each family could live in an apartment; multiple, related families would live in a two-family house or a typical "triple-decker three-family." Starting in the late 1950s, the neighborhood began to change, as second-generation Irish Americans and Italian Americans moved out of Dorchester into the suburbs. Realtors steered African Americans to the area, where low interest loans and modest down payments could afford them a chance for home ownership. Now the streets and homes are filled with black and brown people, some African American, others, like Baron, Puerto Rican.

Baron greeted me from the porch with a wave. I had not seen him for several months since he had been a patient lying in a hospital bed. Back then he was struggling to recover from four stab wounds—one in each leg, one to his abdomen, and another to his chest—and surgery to repair them.

This was the first time I had seen him standing upright. He was thin and looked small beneath his baggy jeans and hooded sweatshirt. His jet-black, curly hair was freshly cut. His skin shined caramel, and except for a small tuft of charcoal hair sprouting from his chin, his face was smooth. Small lines of discomfort and worry showed on his 19-year-old face. Still, he managed a smile when he saw me and motioned me into the house.

The inside of the house was warm and showed none of the weathering of the exterior. The owners of the house had preserved its original detail. The walls were lined with rich mahogany woodwork. Elaborate moldings crowned the ten-foot ceilings. The living room was filled with ornate gilded chairs and two high-backed scarlet sofas, all covered in yellowing vinyl.

It was Sunday, and the house was filled with people. The voices and footsteps of children echoed from upstairs. The strong smell of tobacco smoke floated from the dining room, along with a chorus of Spanish-accented male voices. We walked into the dining room where a small group of men stood at one end of the lace-covered table, smoking and talking and laughing and poking one another on the arm. They stopped abruptly and looked over with an air of expectation.

"This is my uncle. That's his friend. That's my cousin," Baron told me as though we were touring an exhibit. The men smiled without speaking and warmly shook my hand before returning to their banter.

We passed into the warm kitchen, where two women were sitting at the table sipping coffee. The dull, sweet aroma of stewed beans filled the room. "This is my uncle's wife. She is like my mother." He did not introduce me to the other woman, but he said something to both of them in Spanish. His aunt nodded and motioned toward the stairs leading into the basement.

We climbed down the narrow stairs, where the decor suddenly changed again, this time to pollen-yellow pile carpeting and walnut paneling. At the bottom of the stairs, we stood at the beginning of a long hallway that led to a bulkhead door. To the right, there was a room with a mattress lying on the floor. The walls were papered with posters of hip-hop artists. I recognized a few, but most were unfamiliar to me. "This is my room," he told me. "It's like my own little space. I can go outside whenever I want. I don't have to go through the whole house, so it's pretty cool."

We did not go into this room but rather, he walked me halfway down the hall to a small alcove. In it were a small desk, a couple of chairs and a gooseneck lamp.

"We can talk here if it's okay," Baron said.

■ ■ ■

Baron told me that the young man who had attacked him, and whom Baron had been obliged to stab in self-defense, was pressing charges against Baron for assault. Baron was worried about what might happen to him in court.

"Right now, the court's givin' me a lot of problems, you know? They're tryin' to give me two years probation and a record. So I told 'em I want to take it to trial, 'cause I don't want to get probation, and I don't want to have a record. There should be some defense, you know. I mean, they tell me I might have to do six months. Right now, that's one thing I don't want."

Baron shifted in the chair and stretched his right leg out, moaning faintly. "How are you healing up?" I asked him.

"My legs started to improve to a point, but then it just stayed at that one point, and it got skinny. The muscles in my legs, they're kinda shrunk. So every time I try to take steps, or if I'm goin' to take big steps, my leg will just give out on me, and I'll just fall.

"I had a problem one day about a week ago. I was walkin' up the street, and this guy had pulled out a gun. So I tried to run, but I just fell. Turns out the guy was an undercover cop. Some kids were messin' with him, so he pulled out a gun. I didn't know he was a cop. I took two steps and just fell. I always think about that. I mean, what if that was someone else? What if he wasn't a police officer?"

Baron rubbed the leg. "A couple of weeks ago, I got up and my leg was swelled up. It stayed like that for like three days. I couldn't move it. Then it went back down."

He lifted his T-shirt. "I also got a little bump right here," he said, pointing to the scar above his navel. "They tell me it's a stitch and that it will go away in a few months."

Baron slid back into the chair and let out a heavy sigh. "I keep trying to get on with my life, but it seems like I'm going deeper down. Seems like no matter what I try to do, everything crumbles.

"Like, I told you about the nightmares I be havin'. Sometimes I have nightmares about being stabbed all over again. Then other times, I'll have like dreams of, not just being stabbed but being shot or something. I notice that I dream a lot about different stuff."

Baron started to say something but stopped. He looked sheepish. Then he looked me straight in the eye.

"I won't lie to you. The thing that really makes me go to sleep at night? Or that makes the nightmares go away, that helps me knock out? I smoke. I don't even smoke during the day no more.

"I take a little weed, and I'll save it for night. I'll go outside and just smoke it. When I come in the house, the first thing I do is knock out.

"Whenever I don't do that, I get nightmares. Usually when I don't smoke, you'll find me up watchin' TV at like 4 or 5 in the morning. 'Cause I can't sleep.

"That's why I smoke, so I don't think about nothin', and I just go to sleep. But if I don't go to sleep, I think about this problem, that problem, all the problems I have, all the problems that I've been through. I just don't go to sleep."

"Do you smoke more than you used to or less than you used to?" I asked.

"Less," he responded, " 'cause I only smoke at night. I don't worry about the day. I just think about the night. It seems like it's worse at night when I'm by myself."

I was neither surprised nor shocked. Most of the young patients I talked to smoked marijuana, in part to treat their anxiety. In fact, I recalled reading an article about how marijuana and alcohol use soared among New Yorkers in the months following the terrorist attacks on September 11, 2001. Researchers in New York found that people who had true posttraumatic stress disorder or depression were the most likely to increase their use of these drugs. Other researchers have found the same phenomenon in survivors of war or other tragedies. I had never seen such an article about young black men who had been shot or stabbed.

It also did not surprise me that Baron should choose marijuana as his "medication." Unlike the drugs that we prescribed for anxiety, marijuana was readily available in his neighborhood, on his very block. He didn't need to ride the bus or subway to a cold and impersonal building and bare his emotional soul to someone who might easily dismiss his complaints as a thinly veiled attempt to get sleeping pills. He had no health insurance and no primary care doctor, so the option of going to the hospital didn't even occur to him. Instead, he could take a drug with which he was intimately familiar and could adjust how and when he used it to control his symptoms of trauma in his own way.

From what I know, the pharmacological characteristics of marijuana (or, more accurately, its active compound, delta-9-tetrahydrocannabinol, also called THC) made it a logical choice for self-treatment of trauma. At low doses, it can relieve anxiety and create a sense of calm. This was exactly what Baron needed to free him from the images of violence and pain and allow him to go to sleep. He had tested it, and in his mind and his experience, the drug worked.

But I was too well aware of the problems that using a drug in this way could cause him. While at low doses marijuana might provide a sense of calm detachment, at higher doses it could do just the opposite, produce extreme anxiety. Baron, who learned that smoking weed before bed could relieve his nightmares, might smoke more, pushing his dosage higher, on the theory that "more is better." That no two batches of marijuana are alike only made the problem worse. There was no real way for him to control his dosage. He admitted this, telling me that when he smoked too much, he found himself no longer sedate but anxious and paranoid. Added to his already potent symptoms of trauma, I was afraid this effect would plunge him deeper into crisis and isolation.

Marijuana also brought with it the risk of problems with the police, the last thing Baron needed or wanted now. He was already tied up in court. Getting locked up for having a bag of weed would only make that worse. If he was forced to accept probation, he would face frequent and random drug tests. If he failed these tests because of marijuana, he could find himself in jail.

Baron told me that he was also looking for a job that would allow him to get out of the house and give him some money for clothes and to help out his uncle. Since he had only a high school diploma, there were not many places that would hire him. Many of those that would consider him would also ask for a urine drug screen. So his medication of choice, partially effective though it may be, might cut him off from the one thing that he believed would help him get back on his feet: a job.

All of these thoughts ran through me in an instant. At first, I was tempted to do the very thing he was expecting me to do: tell him to stop. But I did not. This was not the time to pry from him the only medicine that gave him relief. Instead, I probed him for other solutions.

"Is there anything that helps you other than smoking weed?"

"Yeah. Sometimes my girl comes to stay with me. Sometimes my cousin stays here, but he just goes to sleep."

"When somebody stays with you, or if your girlfriend stays with you, does that keep you from having nightmares?" I asked.

"Yeah. 'Cause, you know, I've got somebody next to me. I just go to sleep."

I thought we had finished, and I was about to leave when Baron began again. "There's one thing, though, after the whole experience. I started writin' a lot. When I was in the hospital, lying there with nothing to do, I used to write raps. So now I just usually, stay home and write music.

"I do these things all at night. I don't want to go to sleep, you know, 'cause like I told you, I've been getting nightmares and all that. But when I'm up, I can't stop thinking about stuff. So I decided to put 'em down on paper."

"What do you write about?" I asked.

"I just write about things that I see every day or things that I been through or how it is for other people that I know that have been through this."

"You mean that violence has happened to them?"

"Yeah. I think I told you before that I had a friend that got shot. Me and him, we sit sometimes and reminisce about how when you be in the hospital, they won't let you eat, or you couldn't wait to eat. Stuff like that. We talk about stitches and pain, the tubes. I just take all of that and put it into street words."

"All right. So tell me some," I asked.

"Tell you some?"

"Yeah."

"Let me show you." Baron walked back into his bedroom and emerged with a pile of bright yellow ruled papers. He leafed through them and pulled out a page.

"Here is one about the streets: *Yesterday is dead and gone. It's a new day. Dreams of riches on my mind all day and night . . .*" He read deliberately, weaving a poem about someday owning Lexuses and BMWs to display before his friends. He laid out more dreams of "dollar signs" and "lifestyles of the rich and famous" before ending the fantasy by describing himself as "trapped in a street game with no way out."

"That's good," I told him.

Baron looked pleased. "Yeah. To me, it's just fun, you know. I like to do it, especially when I do good, and I look at it. It brings a smile to my face." He added, "When I'm done, I'm gonna get a beat to it. I'm gonna perfect it. . . . I wrote another one about nightmares."

"Can you read it for me?"

This time, he looked embarrassed. "Nah," he said. "You read it yourself. It would be better."

He handed me a folded page and told me, "You can keep it. I have lots of copies of that one."

■ ■ ■

I left the house and walked to my car. My house was not far, just a 10-minute drive, but I didn't feel like driving there just yet. Instead, I sat in my car and watched the autumn wind shake the trees and scatter leaves over the already full gutters.

As I sat, I wondered which was worse: to feel completely numb after horrible trauma, like David, or to be like Baron and feel all the weight of the pain. I know it didn't matter. Each felt trapped in his own way, David searching to find the feelings he had lost and Baron searching for remedies to his constant fear and memory. Baron had found a way to channel his distress by writing raps. He had something to feel good about, even if it took being in the hospital to make space for his art. I wished that somehow David could find something more than the apartment full of empty laughter.

I reached into my breast pocket and pulled out the creased yellow paper. I opened it and read the neatly arranged words. This poem had none of the bravado of Baron's other rhyme. In it, he described how he needed to "stay high" to fight off constant nightmares about his bloody injury and impending legal struggles. The rhyme concluded with this haunting couplet:

Nightmares always seem to turn into reality,
And reality seems to fade into nightmares.

7

ROY IN D.C.

In the fall, I compiled some of the patient stories I had collected and thought how much I had learned from them. I wanted to share some of these insights at the Society of General Internal Medicine annual meeting, where my primary care colleagues gathered to talk about their research. I knew that ordinarily, the topic of violence was rarely touched on, and when it was, it was rarely about situations of violence for young black men. Some presentations there dealt with domestic violence or violence prevention and conflict resolution in schools. I thought there might be space to share some of these stories. A number of people in the organization were doing qualitative research and were using that research to help doctors better understand themselves and their patients. Still, I was unsure if these stories, so complex and filled with violence, would be well received. I wondered if the humanity of the young men on the tapes would simply evaporate when only their voices were there to represent them. I hated the thought that somehow, despite my intentions, I would stigmatize and undermine these young men even further.

The ideas kicked around my head, until finally I cobbled together a proposal for a workshop talk about the stories of these young men. I thought about playing a segment of one of the interviews that might stimulate a conversation about how we, as physicians, could intervene in the lives of these young patients. It seemed like a reasonable idea until I pictured it in my mind. I visualized doctors from Seattle and Houston and Chicago and Miami and New York and even Boston all sitting in a room, speculating about the meaning of what this young man was saying. A few insights might jump out at us, but wouldn't it boil down to a bunch of doctors speculating about a seemingly exotic world that we didn't understand?

At some point it occurred to me that what we needed was the kind of expert who would know more about this than any of us, someone who had lived in and made his way through this world of violence. It made perfect sense to me (if I could pull it off) to take Roy along with me to Washington, D.C., and present him to the audience of doctors as the 23-year-old expert he really was. The idea not only resonated with me, it also made me incredibly hopeful. But I was not sure if Roy would agree to go. He was ambivalent about whether he wanted to become the "poster child" of ex-gang members or to retain the tough identity that had carried him throughout his life up to this point. I asked myself: Would this be a good thing for him to do? Or might the sense that he was being paraded before a fascinated group of strangers make him want to run back to a life that was more real and more familiar, that had nurtured him in the projects?

I remember sitting with him in my office and asking him if he'd be willing to go to Washington, D.C., and spend time talking to these doctors. Money wasn't an issue. I knew that I could get the department to foot the cost of his airfare and hotel. The department would also pick up the incidental costs of food. Roy was typically impassive but agreeable.

"Yeah, why not?" he said. "You know me, I always got something to say."

"But," I pressed, "how would you feel about reacting to a tape of a story without hearing it in advance?" I asked this because I knew that Roy was at his best when he was reacting spontaneously. I didn't want to bring him in as a sort of ringer, as if he were prepped to regurgitate whatever I told him to say. I wanted Roy to be his usual raw, fresh self. I wanted this workshop to be an experiment on how two different worlds could see a problem and focus on it together. Roy was fearless.

"I like it even better that way," he told me.

On the appointed day, Roy and I rode the train to Logan Airport. We passed easily through security in the US Airways terminal and made our way to the gate. As we sat in the waiting area, Roy confessed that he had never been on a plane before. He did not seem particularly excited or anxious about the experience. Certainly, he showed no hint of fear. Instead, he expressed a quiet fascination with the adventure.

I looked at Roy, with his neat fresh cut afro and his pristine construction boots. I couldn't help thinking about how much he had changed in the short time since we walked the ragged path around and around the prerelease building. Through the intervention of one of the CLUB's benefactors who saw the promise in Roy, he had landed a paid internship in the office of John Kerry. He was working as an office assistant, a role possibly beneath his intellect and skill set. But given that just months earlier, he had been locked up for a violent crime, this position seemed nothing short of a miracle.

"You excited about the job in the senator's office?" I asked, projecting my own enthusiasm.

"Yeah, pretty much," he replied, nodding and flashing a wry smile. He said no more and seemed content to examine the columns of frantic travelers talking too loud on their cell phones and clutching their plastic water bottles.

They called our flight. After we boarded, Roy settled into the window seat on the Boeing 737. He peered out the window as the airliner sped down the runway for takeoff. I thought back to my first flight and remembered the odd mixture of fear and exhilaration. I could see the same emotions in Roy's eyes as the plane lifted off the runway. Even as it did, he seemed to relax as though he were floating above the chaos that was Boston. The flight attendant brought us sodas and peanuts, and we chatted. Roy seemed to forget that we were floating at 32,000 feet.

We got into Washington and took a cab to the Marriott Hotel in Crystal City, Virginia. We checked into a room that looked out at the district; the Washington Monument was a brilliant white against the tangerine-gray twilight sky. We ordered room service and unabashedly munched on oversized Marriott hamburgers and hand-cut French fries. Roy ordered a Heineken and a glass of ice and, quirkily, had his beer on the rocks. We whiled away the evening watching the Chicago Bulls beat up on the Cleveland Cavaliers in the NBA playoffs. Roy analyzed the game passionately, picking apart why a given play didn't work and why the Cavs were destined to lose.

The next day, when the time came for the workshop, I felt nervous and excited, but Roy seemed completely calm. He dressed in a preppy-looking ivory wool sweater with a neck framed by red and blue. I joked with him that he was wearing the colors of the American flag, and he laughed. We made our way down through the hotel lobby and into the adjoining convention center. All around us, hyperactive researchers in business attire rushed toward various sessions, many of them carrying long tubes holding their poster presentations. Others strolled with their heads buried in the conference program, oblivious to anyone around them. Outside of each presentation room was an easel holding a sign announcing the topic of the session. We worked our way around the hallways until we found the sign for "Understanding Violence in Young Black Men."

The room was filled with rows of gilded chairs. A table set up in the front held several microphones and sweaty pitchers of ice water. We took our places at the table as the room began to fill with doctors and researchers from all over the country, a disproportionate number of them physicians of color. Eventually, a diverse group of about 15 people settled into the seats, looking intrigued to see Roy sitting at the front of the room.

I began by describing why I felt it was important to understand the lives and experiences of young black men who had been injured. I then introduced Roy, who sat straight-faced and relaxed, as the expert who would help us interpret what we would hear. I hooked up the speaker and began to play the tape, projecting the young man's deep voice throughout the room. The people in the room squinted and concentrated, trying to make out the nuances of the voice. Roy also turned his eyes up toward the ceiling and listened intently.

The young man on the tape—we called him Tony—told the story of getting stabbed in a fight in Roxbury. This 23-year-old man narrated how he went into a pizza shop in his neighborhood and ran into a guy with whom he had had a past "beef." They began to argue, and the words grew from nasty to threatening. Finally, the young man beckoned Tony outside to fight, but first he flashed a knife. Tony reached over the counter, grabbed a butcher knife, and bolted outside to brawl. But when Tony walked out the door, the other young man hit him in the head with a brick, and the blood from the wound ran into his eyes, blinding him and causing him to drop his knife. The assailant and his friends chased Tony, stabbing him several times before he got away. Tony fled toward his home and up the steps of his father's brownstone. As he recounted in the interview, "I rang the doorbell for my father to come down. When he came to the door, I told him to take my clothes off because the ambulance people be cutting up your clothes." Tony's voice on the tape went on to confess that he had hidden several vials of crack cocaine under his tongue. When he saw the police cars arrive at his house, he swallowed them. Tony told how the cocaine entered his system and, in combination with his injuries, almost killed him. He ended his story with the statement: "Guess it's from being in the wrong place at the wrong time." The tape played for just four minutes until he reached this final pronouncement, and I turned off the tape.

Immediately Roy began to speak, explaining what he thought was happening from his perspective. His eagerness to get his thoughts out caught me off guard. I touched Roy on his arm. "Roy, since you are here as the expert, how about we let folks in the audience respond first and ask any questions they might have? Then you can respond with your ideas." Roy sat back looking slightly frustrated but nodded as if to say he would go along with my suggestion.

An older man with a salt-and-pepper beard stood up and expressed confusion about why Tony would have engaged in an argument so easily. Why couldn't he just walk away? A younger woman with olive skin, whose physique suggested that she was in the early stages of pregnancy, marveled that the young man seemed more concerned about his clothing than the fact of being stabbed within an inch of his life. Roy listened closely to each question, most of which seemed cautiously framed, as though by asking about the motives of the man on the tape the speakers might offend an entire tribe, of which Roy was a member. When he began to answer, Roy did not sound offended by the questions, but his voice carried its usual edge of challenge, sometimes carried along by rhetorical questions.

"This guy learned a totally different set of rules than the ones you learned growing up," he told them. "They are the same rules I learned. You ask why he is so worried about his clothes. What else does he have to look forward to? His clothes might be one of the few things in this world that he's proud of. The sad part is that he has seen so many people get shot up that he knows exactly what's gonna happen when the ambulance gets there, if it actually comes. And they will cut off your clothes: that is real." Roy continued in a preaching tone. "And I know we all wanna judge the fact that this guy was selling crack. That's of course why he had the rocks under his tongue. To you, because y'all are doctors and all that, it might seem like a bad decision. But that's because you have lots of options and income and chances to make your life mean something. For him, selling crack is all he can see. So in the end, we can preach at people not to sell drugs, but they will only stop selling drugs when they see a better way to go. That's what happened to me. I let the drug-selling thing go when I had something better.

"Now I know y'all are thinking, 'Oh no, he did not just tell us that he used to sell drugs,' but I did. And in a lot of ways, selling drugs was easier than having a regular job. Even though I am on the right path, I have to tell myself every day that even though being good is a whole lot harder than being bad, I have to do good."

Just as I had hoped, Roy laid things out bluntly and confidently. In doing so, I could see him regaining the confidence that he displayed every day in Boston. He peppered the audience with questions, and they nodded with abashed understanding at the explanations he offered.

Though the session was slated to last an hour, it drifted over as more people queried Roy about what he thought the solutions to violence were. After the session officially ended, several people came up to congratulate Roy for his courage in being there. Roy accepted the compliments, but he did so with ambivalence, again resisting the role as "poster boy" for people who had "turned their lives around." Both of us left feeling that we had done something new and strong and powerful, although Roy said little about the session itself.

■ ■ ■

The next day we went downstairs to the mall connected to the Marriott and found the food court so that we could grab breakfast before heading out to do a lightning tour of D.C. We stopped at a small deli grill and ordered egg sandwiches on English muffins. We stood chatting as the short-order cook cracked the eggs onto the grill several yards away and began to manipulate them with a large spatula. As he did, I noticed that he was using the same spatula to flip our eggs that he was using to cook the raw chicken on a nearby grill. He could easily be contaminating our sandwiches with salmonella, as the bacteria were undoubtedly coating the raw chicken. I turned to Roy and shook my head. "He's contaminating our food with that spatula."

"So, cuss him out," Roy instructed matter-of-factly.

Roy was serious. For Roy it wouldn't be enough just to tell the cook that he was making a mistake; it had to be said in a particular way.

"No," I told him. "I am not going to cuss him out, but we are not going to eat those sandwiches, either." I called the cashier over and asked for the cook's attention. I explained to him that he was risking making us sick by the way he was using the spatula. He immediately admitted his mistake and apologized. He discarded the eggs and the bread and started again, this time using perfect technique. He gave the sandwiches to us without charge. Still, Roy glared at him as we walked over to a nearby table.

"It's cool, man. I think he just made a mistake."

"Are you tellin' me that dude doesn't know about salmonella? Isn't it his job to know?" Roy fired back. "I woulda cussed the dude out. That way he'll remember the next time."

"You think?" I asked with my own skepticism.

"Yeah. I know that's not you, but that's how I am. I just can't let things go like that. I guess I was just bred to be confrontational."

We sat and ate our sandwiches and sipped our hot coffees. Despite the early hour, many people, young and old, were milling about the mall. A small group of young African American men passed. Roy locked eyes with them and tracked them as they walked away. The menacing glare they exchanged evaporated after a long moment, and then Roy looked back to me.

"What was that about?" I asked Roy.

"What?" he asked.

"The staring."

"Yeah. That's just me," Roy said. "I got an eye problem."

"An eye problem?"

"That's how I grew up. I just look at people. I can't help it. When somebody looks at me, I just have to keep looking at them until they look away. Sometimes it causes trouble, but most of the time, they just look away, and we go on about our business.

"You know how I told you that my parents taught me how to fight and how to do crime?"

"Yeah, you did."

"So while other parents were teaching their kids to play baseball and coaching their soccer teams, my parents were teaching us how to beat up other people's kids."

"Didn't you say that your mother went to bat for you to get you transferred out to the school in Lincoln?"

Roy shook his head as if to dispute this but then acknowledged, "Yeah, she did that much. But ain't that what parents are supposed to do?"

Roy shifted in his seat and bounced his shoulders as he spoke. His agitation brought forth the strong twang of his Boston accent. "I don't think I told you how I really got into the streets. I was living with my moms, 'cause her and my father weren't together. She lived over on Seaver down behind the park." Roy's accent held onto the last word so that it emerged as *pahk*.

"She was living with this dude, and we didn't really get along. So one day I came home and he says to me, 'You didn't take out the trash before you left.' So I just stood there looking at him like, 'So? You couldn't take it out yourself?'

"So he says, 'I'm going to have to punish you.' So I looked back at him like, 'First of all, you ain't my father. And you want me to take out the trash? Fine.' So I walked out and took out the trash, and I kept going."

"How old were you?" I asked.

"Twelve. I remember because I was already at Lincoln. This was the summer, though."

"So, where did you go?"

"I went up around the block up on Elm Hill and Sonoma where my brother and his friends used to hang out. I was hanging around with all these older dudes who were out on the block dealing. I hung with them all day. So finally they say, 'Hey kid, isn't it time for you to run home?'

"I just stayed there like, 'No, this is where I am gonna hang.' So after a while they was like, 'This young'n is serious.' So they just rolled me into their business.

"There was this other young kid named Manny. Me and him were lookouts. We would go up on the roof and keep an eye out for the cops. Manny's mother was an alcoholic, and he was never sure when she would be home. Sometimes she was so knocked out that it was 3 or 4 in the morning before he could get inside. So we would be out in the street all night. Sometimes we would sleep up on the roof."

Roy shook his head and chuckled with disgust. "Little kids just doing crime.

"Finally one day, I'm up on the roof, and the cops sweep through. And they scoop up all my friends. So they're all locked up, and I'm out there alone.

"So I started to sleep up at the top of the stairwell in the projects where my father lived." Roy paused and then sighed heavily. "Something else, and I don't think I've told this to many people. Maybe just a couple of people ever. But that summer when we couldn't stay with Manny's mother 'cause she was too drunk to wake up, we had to find someplace else to sleep. So you know up in Franklin Park where the old zoo used to be? You know those old bear cages? Well, we used to go up and sleep there."

I knew the place Roy was talking about. Several mornings a week, I would get up with the sun, put on warm gear and run the half-mile or so from my house to the park. Then I would follow the few miles of trail around the tranquil golf course in the center of the meadow. Franklin Park was an unusually beautiful and almost undiscovered urban oasis, designed by Frederick Law Olmsted, the same landscape architect who created Central Park in New York.

It was only after running there for years that I strayed from my usual route and followed a path up the hill behind School-boy Stadium. Halfway up the hill, I came upon the crumbling relics. At first the site looked like an abandoned fortress, but as

I shuffled past I realized that these were in fact animal cages. These were the remains of the old zoo, long since relocated to the south side of the park. Thick bars remained anchored to decaying slabs of concrete, and weeds had taken over the space. It would have felt ominous even if it had not once housed captive bears. It had never occurred to me that these long-abandoned manmade caves might once have served as a makeshift bedroom for young boys like Roy.

Roy shook his head as if he could not believe this had been his life. "So after my friends got locked up, I slept up there sometimes. But mostly I would sleep up in the stairway at my Pop's place.

"After a few weeks of being out there by myself, I was just so tired. My legs were aching. I just knew I had to get off the streets. So I went to my father's house, and I knocked on the door. And he came out like it was nothing, like he had been seeing me the whole time. And when I told him where I was living and how I got there, we just both broke down."

Roy paused and lowered his head as his eyes filled up. He tore gently at the foil that had enveloped the breakfast sandwich. He resumed letting a bold tear flow freely down his cheek. "After that I just went to sleep. I must have slept for like three days straight. I don't even remember getting up to eat.

"The thing that woke me up was the sound of my mother's voice arguing with my father. So she came into the room where I was sleeping and I got up. Like I told you, my mom is tough. So she just hauled off and hit me. And she had all this jewelry on her hands so she really marked me."

Roy stopped and shrugged. I don't think either of us anticipated that my question about his staring match with the passersby would take us down this road. We both sat with the silence for a moment before Roy piped up, "So that's my family."

I just nodded and took it in. I wondered how I could have known Roy for two years and only now hear of this significant trauma in his life. Roy had not been shot or stabbed, like the other young men I have talked to. But he labored under a different kind of weight, and now it was bleeding slowly through his hard exterior.

Roy broke the pensive silence. "So the whole philosophy that I grew up with was this: winning justifies everything. That was it. Everything I have seen in my life is based on that. And in a way, I kind of think it's true. Not just in the projects, but you see it all the time—in politics, in business, in sports—that's the idea: winning justifies everything!"

He paused to sip the lukewarm coffee before saying matter-of-factly, "I kind of think that it gave me a warped sense of what's right and what's wrong."

Roy rocked back in his chair. He had a way of summing things up, encapsulating painful truths as though summing them up prevented them from damaging him. At first, I thought that it was his way of rebuffing further exploration, but I came to understand it as his own ability to accept events, even painful ones, without feeling intensely sorry for himself. If I had not known him for this long, I might have taken this as callousness or indifference. But it was not that. It was part of what made Roy unique.

"You ready?" Roy asked.

"Sure," I said.

We cleared the table of our half-eaten sandwiches and set out into the bright sunlight. We boarded the Metro train and rode it across the Potomac. Through the dusty subway windows, we both pointed out the familiar landmarks and negotiated which of them Roy wanted to see.

We started on the Mall and strode the distance from the Washington Monument to the Lincoln Memorial. We stood in different spots to see which vantage point best recreated the camera's view of Martin Luther King Jr. as he gave his "I Have a Dream" speech. I took Roy's photo as he leaned against the glassy wall of the Vietnam Memorial. Around the back of the White House, Roy perched himself against the wrought iron fence, folded his arms across his chest, and asked me to take his picture. Just as I snapped the shutter, he extended his middle finger from where it lay on his arm. (Later, this rebellious pose would be the only snapshot he would request in a print.) The few hours passed quickly. The childlike side of Roy that emerged was hyperfriendly to almost every fellow tourist. In the safety of this new experience, he eagerly wrapped himself in this new community.

Out on the Mall, we met a young man from Los Angeles who was there with a church group. I thought that he and Roy would have had little in common, but they eagerly connected and talked about their respective cities, the police, girls, and what they both liked about D.C. In the end, they pledged to keep in touch, but I do not think they did. For Roy, this moment was like the pleasant dream that precedes a nightmare— seeming all the more unreal after the terror of the bad dream has bruised it.

8

KARI IN THE CLINIC

When I saw Kari a week after he was released from the hospital, he was walking slowly toward the clinic building. He had come back to see the surgeon who had repaired the wounds in his chest and abdomen. But he had also agreed to meet me so that we could talk more about what he had gone through.

Trying to guard his abdomen against pain, Kari walked stiffly and bent over, like an old man. As he walked, he threw each leg out in front of him with a slight twist so that his upper body wobbled each time he planted a heel into the pavement. Another young man walked beside Kari, shepherding him with outstretched hands but careful not to touch him. He held his hands out, framing Kari in order to catch him should he tumble over.

"It's good to see you," I said.

"Good to be seen," Kari said smiling. "I'm better, but not all the way there." He motioned toward the young man next to him. "This is my friend Marlon." His friend was lanky with dreadlocks that flowed down his face to join the African leather beads hanging around his neck. Marlon shook my hand.

"He's into music, and he's real good," Kari told me. "He just got a record contract. Like $80,000, man." A rich smile spread across Marlon's face.

"Wow. Congratulations," I said.

Kari chimed in, "We're gonna open a recording studio together."

Marlon laid his hand on Kari's shoulder in agreement.

"It'll be good. Give him something to do," Marlon said.

We walked through the lobby and past long lines of customers at the pharmacy and at the new coffee kiosk. The earthy aroma of coffee thrown off by the new and bustling Dunkin' Donuts filled the lobby space and seemed out of place in the aging structure. Kari shuffled along, occasionally wincing in pain, but mostly he looked as though he'd gotten used to walking this way. Marlon and I flanked him, matching his pace by walking with conspicuous slowness.

The elevator took us to the third floor, and we strolled to the surgical clinic. The waiting room, as usual, was brimming with patients, a consequence of the fact that all patients were told to arrive at 9 a.m. Harried clerks behind the desk thrust clipboards at the crush of patients in front of them, plopped Bic pens onto the cold white sheets of paper. I scanned the patients in the waiting room. An elderly black woman hobbled to the desk to return her form. I could not tell whether her slow, pained gait was a result of a recent operation or whether she was here seeking relief for something that caused her to walk this way.

But what most struck me was that almost half of the patients there were young men—some black, some Latino, and a few white—who limped up to the desk in a way that told me they had been wounded. Kari joined the rest of these young men in the line, content to let the overwhelmed clerks go through their chaotic routine. Marlon stood at Kari's side, still guarding him as if he were delivering an important parcel to its final destination. I leaned against the wall and watched this action, just as it played out every day. My clinic down the hall seemed placid by comparison. But I recognized that many of my patients in the Young Men's Health Clinic had made a stop in this clinic, too. At least once a session, a patient lifted his shirt to reveal the delicate scars that had been tended to here.

After nearly twenty minutes, Kari and Marlon returned from the desk. Kari told me, "They say it's gonna be at least an hour, maybe more." Neither he nor Marlon seemed troubled by having to wait. Marlon appeared fascinated by all the faces and activity. Kari, on the other hand, looked glad to be out of the house.

"Why don't we find a quiet place to talk?" I asked Kari.

"Sure," Kari said, immediately turning to Marlon.

"I'll hang here, in case they call you," Marlon said. "I'm cool."

Kari and I walked halfway down the hall to where the diabetes clinic normally met. It was an off day for this clinic, so the hallway was deserted and all the rooms were free. We chose a space, leaving the door ajar in case the surgeons moved through the crowd of patients more quickly than anticipated.

Kari looked different than he looked that day when the nurse dressed his wound. Gone was the matted hair of the hospital room, replaced by a crisp razor cut. At 18, his round face was still childlike. His teeth were a shocking white against his brown lips. His skin was smooth and almost jet-black.

But when I looked closer, I could still see the telltale crack on the lips of the right side of his mouth, a remnant of the plastic tube that ran from the breathing machine, across his tongue, and into his lungs. He sat slightly hunched over, and when he spoke, he turned his head to me but his body remained strangely still, an attempt to avoid the pain brought on by sudden movement. The whites of his eyes were glazed and pale. His pupils had constricted to pin points, a side effect of the opiates he was taking for pain.

Kari seemed less anxious to tell his story than to understand why I wanted to hear it. "So you wanna hear the whole thing? Like from the beginning?"

"Whatever you want to talk about. Start where you want to start," I said.

"Well, I was comin' from Dorchester High, 'cause my boy, Rod, he got a car and he think his sound system in his car is louder than anyone else's. So he was blastin' his music. But the cops came and told us that we had to turn the music down.

"So that's when he went to drop me off. I was gonna go home, but I do not know why I didn't just stop and go home. For some reason, he drove right past my house, and I got out up the street. I guess I just didn't tell him to stop in time.

"So I was walkin' back up the block to my house, and I seen the dude from a distance on a bike. He rode up on me acting casual, like it wasn't nothin'. So he stops right in front of me and says, 'Run that.'"

"What does that mean?" I asked.

"Oh," said Kari, as if he suddenly remembered that I might not understand what he meant. "'Run that' means he wanted to take my chain.

"So I just looked at him, and I seen that he had his hand in his pocket, like he was holdin' his gun. I just tried to push him, and he fell off the bike. So I tried to run, and he started shootin'. I guess he was layin' on the ground shootin'.

"I think it was the second shot or the third shot that hit me in my back, 'cause I felt it as soon as it went in. One side of my body just went numb. I remember my arm goin' like this and I couldn't pull it down."

Kari grimaced slightly as he raised his right arm to demonstrate. He held his arm out parallel to the ground with his hand hanging down toward the floor.

"Then my leg went back, and I couldn't pull it out. So I was just layin' there on the ground. That's when he ran up on me. He said 'I should kill you.'

"He didn't even snatch my chain off my neck. He just lightly took it off. Then he patted my pocket like that and reached in my pocket and took fifty dollars outta my pocket. Then he just ran. He left like three dollars in my pocket."

Kari paused as if he had reached the end of his story. I paused with him, not wanting to push him too much. He raised his eyebrows.

"You want to hear more?"

"Yep. Again, as much as you want to talk about."

"Oh," Kari said, looking slightly puzzled. He squinted, concentrating hard to pull up the details. He then began to speak slowly, like he was reconstructing a dream or a scene from a television action drama.

I recognized in this the look of someone telling a story for the first time. My guess was that in the week or so since he had been shot, Kari had told the story about the young gunman on the bike many times when friends and family asked, "What happened?" But the part of his story that dealt with the moments on the ground and the ride to the hospital and the trauma in the emergency room was not what the curious friends tended to ask about.

I also sensed that in order to tell this, he had to draw on the memories that were recorded by his brain after the bullets had penetrated his flesh. The threat of injury caused his body to leap to rapid preparation for a response, causing his adrenal glands to release a surge of catecholamines—hormones like adrenaline and cortisol that regulate the body's protective "fight or flight" response. These chemicals allowed him to resist and to get up after being shot. They blunted the pain momentarily so that he could try to escape and get help from his friends and neighbors. At the same time, the chemicals changed how memory was processed and recorded, sometimes rendering memories sharper and more vivid, other times suppressing them from his conscious memory altogether. Kari struggled to piece together the scene from the fragments in his memory.

"Well, I was layin' on the ground. It took the ambulance a real long time to come. My friend poured a soda on my back. Then the ambulance came." He stopped for a second but continued to concentrate intensely. "I don't know. I thought I was gonna die, though. I really did. I really did."

"You said your friend poured a soda on your back?" I asked wondering if I had heard him right.

"Yeah."

"What was that about?"

" 'Cause I was on the ground and I just kept sayin' I was hot and it was burnin'. He thought I was paralyzed, 'cause my legs just kept like shakin' real, real fast." Kari's voice became halting and frustrated. "I don't know. He was hysterical. He just poured the soda on my back. I didn't feel it, though."

Kari looked up, trying to capture the details as they flashed through his mind. Still, he moved through each piece of the story, piecing together the chaotic details as best he could.

"I got up and I started walkin', and everybody was like, 'Lay down! Lay down!' They was tellin' me that the bullet was gonna travel. That was gettin' me scared.

"Then the cops came, but they wasn't even doin' me no favors either. No help or nothin'. They wouldn't let my man touch me. They was like, 'Leave him alone. Don't touch him.'

"And this one police officer was standin' over me sayin', 'Don't do nothin' stupid. Don't do nothin' stupid, like die.' That made me so mad.

"And then, another police car came up the street, doin' like a hundred. He seen me layin' in the middle of the street, and he just stopped right in front of me, inches from my head. All the dirt, rocks, everything was in my mouth and my eyes." He shuddered at the memory.

"I was shook. I was scared. I was really scared." He stuck out his tongue as if he were trying to rid himself of a bad taste.

"How about getting to the hospital?" I asked.

"The ambulance driver was crazy. I don't know what he was thinkin'. He was goin' mad slow until he hit the corners, then it seemed like he was speedin' up. The doctors that was in the back, tryin' to work on me, they was all fallin', screamin' at him, everything. That was the longest ambulance ride! I'm askin', 'Where we goin? What hospital am I goin' to?' It seemed like I was in that ambulance for hours."

Kari paused again to think. Suddenly his face brightened as he hooked onto a detail. "When I got to the hospital, this doctor was there. He was good. I don't even know his name. Who's the doctor that wears the glasses?" he asked, now pressing me for the details to fill in his memory. "He wears red glasses? He's like, younger."

"What else does he look like?" I asked.

"He's skinny. He's kinda tall. He's a white guy. He wears a stretch band around the back of his head for his glasses."

Kari strained to give me these very specific details, like he was describing a person standing in front of him. But still, except for the stretch band for his glasses, this generic description could have fit most of the male physicians in the hospital. I searched my mind to see if I could think of one who wore such a strap, but I came up empty.

"There are a lot of doctors," I conceded, "so I'm not sure which one you mean. But tell me about him."

"Well, when I got to the hospital, he made me feel a lot better, 'cause he was holdin' my hand and he kept tellin' me, 'Just hold on. You're gonna be all right. I ain't gonna let you die.'

"He just kept tellin' me that. He made me feel a lot better, a lot better.

" 'Cause I remember them takin' the X-rays, when I was bleeding. And when they turned me to take X-rays, it was hurting. There was like five doctors there, and all of 'em was pushin' on my stomach. They didn't even take me right to surgery. They just kept takin' more X-rays.

"I was heated. I was mad.

"Then, after like a half an hour, they brought me to the operating room. They put that thing on my face, and it felt like they was smothering me.

"Next thing I knew, I was waking up the next day with mad tubes in my mouth and my nose, both sides of my chest. Tubes were everywhere, man. That was the thing that hurt the most, I think: the aftereffects from all the tubes. That was crazy."

I remembered seeing Kari just as he described. But I was

struck by how much of what I had come to accept as normal in the course of saving a life, he interpreted as malicious. It had never occurred to me that a young patient in pain who had never before seen the inside of an operating room would interpret the mask that delivers life-sustaining oxygen as an instrument intended to suffocate him. All of the tubes that made it possible for him to breathe and to avoid infection seemed to him to be more menacing than the bullet that put him there.

No wonder the rift between caregivers and injured patients was so wide. Nothing was more hurtful to caregivers than being accused of trying to hurt someone they were actually trying to help. But in this case, I doubted that any of the caregivers had the time to explain to Kari the purpose of the strange implements being thrust at him and into him.

"And then I was in intensive care. I felt they was doin' their job good. Then, when I moved down to the other floor, I don't think half the nurses knew what they was doin'. I mean, they probably knew what they was doin', but they weren't on their job like they're supposed to.

"I remember one morning when I was down there, I was layin' in my throw-up for like half an hour. And the surgeon, the doctor that was holdin' my hand? He came in my room and cleaned up my throw-up. The nurse told me it wasn't her job to come clean it up. I was laying *in it*. It was all over me, on my sheets and everything. I was so mad. I was mad there. Mad."

As much as I wanted to believe that a doctor cleaned his bed and changed his sheets, I knew that Kari had gotten this part wrong. Most of us doctors didn't even know where the sheets were kept, much less how to change them. Most would have called a nurse to clean up the mess before even examining the patient. As a doctor, it pained me to admit it, but it was the truth. I suspected that Kari, having little experience with the world of doctors and nurses, made the assumption that any male provider was a doctor and any female, a nurse. But since the kind nurse did not explain that he was in fact a male nurse, his helpful actions were not credited to the nursing profession.

Sadly, coupled with Kari's misunderstanding that a nurse had answered his call button (it was more likely a unit clerk), Kari came away with a negative impression of nurses overall.

Kari sighed and shook his head. "I wouldn't want to go back to the hospital again, man. Never again. Never."

"That sounds really rough," I said.

"Man, you don't even know. But this whole thing changed my life, I think. Even though somethin' bad happened, I think somethin' good happened out of it too. You know?"

"Tell me more."

Kari shifted and pulled at his shirt like he too was trying to figure out what he meant. "I think it was a wake-up call for me. I think that God just knew I had to get my life together and do somethin' different.

"I got a son, and I wasn't spendin' time with him. Even though I did what I had to do and made sure he had everything he needed, I really never spent time with him and stuff. Now I see what I was missin' out on. You know what I mean?

"See, my father was never around, and he never did anything for me. So I need to make sure my son knows I'm with him. I gotta spend as much time as I can with him. Now, I know I have to be a good father. That's like, mandatory.

"Before, I was taking it lightly. But now I feel like that coulda been my last day on this earth. Really, it just coulda been.

"The doctors keep tellin' me I'm real lucky. I coulda been paralyzed, or I coulda died. They said one bullet was three inches away from my spine, two inches away from my heart. They can't believe it came that close.

"When it's time, when God wants me to come, He's gonna take me. So if He don't want me to come yet, I shouldn't be worried. You know? I believe I just wasn't ready to go, 'cause I wasn't at peace with myself. I would have went to hell."

Kari sighed deeply. "So I plan to try to straighten everything out, be at peace with myself. I think I will be all right."

"So tell me how else being shot has changed your life."

"I just look at life totally different now. Like family-wise, I think I care more about my family than I did before. I want to be around 'em more. To be honest, before, I was kind of a stingy dude. But now, I give more, you know?

" 'Cause I might not be here. Any day, I could be gone—by accident, whatever."

Kari paused and then looked up past me, over my shoulder and through the partially open door. I turned and saw Marlon, who had found us after searching several hallways. He told us it was time for Kari to see the surgeons. It felt like an odd place to pause, but we had no choice but to leave this conversation for later. Marlon and I walked Kari back up the hall and left him in the hands of a nurse, who escorted him into an exam room.

Kari was with the surgeon for less than twenty minutes; we were surprised to see him emerge so soon. "They say I'm healing good for somebody who got shot a week ago," he told us. "They gave me some more pain medicine and this sheet to get physical therapy. But they say I ain't ready for that yet." He seemed satisfied with the news that the surgeons were satisfied. "I gotta come back in a couple of weeks. That's it."

We walked back toward the elevators and rode back down to the lobby. A long line of patients snaked from the pharmacy and spilled into the lobby. Kari looked toward the crowd. "I can't stand in that line. I'll get this up the street from me."

We walked outside and stood again on the plaza where we had met earlier. We were shaking hands to say goodbye when I saw Laura, a motherly middle-aged African American woman who, until recently, worked in the office of one of the busiest trauma surgeons here. She was walking up the path to the entrance, carrying the McDonald's bag that held her lunch. She walked right up to us and greeted us boldly.

"Hey, Dr. Rich. Are these your patients?" I did not know what to make of the question or her reason for wanting to know. At first, I thought she must have known Kari and Marlon and that she simply wanted to emphasize the connection.

I answered her: "No, they're my colleagues." It was an awkward response, but it would have been improper for me to tell her that they were my patients. She persisted.

"Well, I hope you keep them on the straight and narrow. 'Cause you know, there are lots of young men up there in the clinic, getting shot and stabbed, and we just have to make it stop. They are out there gangbanging, and they don't even care that they can lose their lives. I'm prayin' for y'all," she said, looking at Kari and Marlon. "But you know, God only helps those that help themselves."

I was surprised that she was going on this way without knowing anything about Kari and Marlon. I looked at them, but they did not seem bothered. They wore sheepish smiles on their faces and listened as though they were no strangers to speeches like this one, full of earnest exhortations from a surrogate mother anxious to make these problems go away.

"These young men are doing well. You don't have to worry," I said, hoping this would satisfy her. She finished her exhortations with a smile and a sharp nod, as if she had given them just the pep talk they needed. It was apparent that in her mind, she was simply making pleasant small talk, but in reality, she had presumed to know their lives.

"See you, Dr. Rich," she said and swept into the building.

I turned to Kari and Marlon to apologize. "I'm sorry. That wasn't right."

"I didn't feel like she was talkin' about us," Kari said. "Maybe her kid is doin' bad."

Marlon nodded. "A lot of kids out here are gettin' killed, so she's not wrong."

"You may be right," I said. Both he and Kari seemed unbothered. I was impressed with their generosity toward her.

Kari was walking more slowly now and grimacing as he shifted his weight back and forth from one foot to the other. "Are you going to be all right on the bus?" I asked.

"No, we're gonna take a cab home," Marlon interjected.

"Yeah, too much walking today," Kari added.

A taxi with a red, white, and blue logo pulled up, and Kari slowly climbed in the back. "Thanks, Doc," he called from inside.

"No, thank *you*," I answered as Marlon slid into the cab and pulled the door closed. "We'll talk soon."

9

MARK IN THE NEIGHBORHOOD

One summer evening a few months later, I pulled up in front of a tired two-story house on a street just off Wheatland Avenue. The day was still bright, even though it was almost 7 p.m. The small street was only about five miles from my home in Roxbury, but I had never been on this street before. Unlike the other homes on the block, this one was set back from the curb, separated from the other houses by a small alley. The front yard was scattered with debris, and there were cats all around. A black dog ran at me and barked from behind a wire fence. I was startled but kept walking, trying not to look at him. As I continued walking to the house, I passed two abandoned cars that were sitting in the yard, one of which had all the windows broken out.

I rang the bell several times before Mark stuck his head out of the second-floor window.

"I am going to throw you down the keys," he told me.

He tossed down the keys, and I unlocked both the top and bottom bolts. The door swung open into a dark vestibule. The air smelled of cat urine, and there was the faint odor of gas, as if the pilot light in a stove had gone out. I started up, and he met me halfway, propped up on crutches. He was shirtless and wearing a pair of basketball shorts. His right leg was in a heavy black brace, and there were bandages underneath it running from his knee to his groin. Nonetheless, he moved well on the crutches and bounced up the stairs in front of me to his apartment.

The door to his apartment had no knob, just a round opening where the knob should have been. To keep the door closed, Mark had looped a piece of cloth through the hole. He motioned me inside, then closed the door and braced it with a wooden stick and the metal rail from a bed frame.

"I don't feel safe here," he told me, "but this is where I live now."

The apartment was bright but mostly empty. We walked back through a small dark kitchen and into a side bedroom where there was a mattress on the floor. Mark eased himself down onto it, carefully guarding his right leg and wincing with pain. The floor was stacked with papers and videotapes piled up against the windows. A nearby shelf and a rolling desk chair held heaps of clothing. On another chair there was a television; on the floor, a stereo.

Out of nowhere, two slate-gray cats appeared and he beckoned them to him. They walked across his chest. As we talked, he rubbed them and scratched their heads.

Mark was 25, but he looked younger. His hair was straight black with just a hint of a curl. His skin was the color of coffee with half a spoonful of cream, and his body was lean. As he propped himself up on his elbows on the mattress, his ribs showed through the skin on his chest. He pinched at his belly with disgust.

"I lost a lot of weight being sick. I gotta bulk back up. Can't even defend myself now. My leg is all fucked up. And I'm alone here.

"Just the other night, somebody came and busted out the windows in my car. I could hear them doin' it, but I couldn't do nothing about it. I'm thinking they might come back here and try to fuck me up. What am I gonna do, all crippled like this?"

I thought back to the vandalized car that I had passed in the yard on my way in. I had assumed it was an abandoned car, not too unusual a sight in Dorchester in those days. My own car sat just a few yards away.

"That day just changed my whole life," Mark said.

"Tell me about that."

"It was a nice day. I was drinkin' Heinekens. I was playing basketball, and I kept on stealin' the ball from this one dude. So he called me a drunk-ass bitch. I told him, 'I ain't no bitch. I might be a drunk ass, but I ain't no bitch.'

"I didn't even know the guy from Adam. That's why I was so shocked when he called me a drunk-ass bitch.

"And then he pushed me. So I punched him dead square in his face. He was a big guy. And I was by myself. I guess he was with his friends. And one of his friends, I guess, hit me over the head wit' a bottle and stabbed me in the neck.

"Once that happened, I just turned around and started running, tryna get up outta the situation. As soon as I started runnin', I heard gunshots, like thirty or forty. I don't know how many.

"One thing I do know is that I'm just barely livin' today, you know? Got shot in the artery, got three screws in my knee. Can't walk on it. This leg's messed up. And the worst part is that I got shot over nothin'. Me and the guy got in a fight. We stopped fightin'. It was supposed to be done, you know? But his people took it to another level."

"What happened next, after you got shot?" I asked.

"I don't remember much about that. Woke up in the ICU. They told me I had a strong will. They said I lost a lotta blood, so they asked my permission to give me blood transfusions. I had like three bags of blood. Now I got somebody else's blood in me.

"I don't know how it happened like that. I don't even know why. I wasn't supposed to get shot. Not me! Maybe years ago, when I was bein' bad and stuff, you know, but I've been tryin' to change my life around and do right things. Before I got shot I was working, doing construction. So, I mean, I've been tryin' to turn my life around, and this just put a little dark spot on my life right now."

"When you said you were 'being bad' in the past, what do you mean?"

"Bein' bad in the streets, doin' whatever it takes. Anything and everything. And I figured that this here shoulda happened to me when I was doin' all that crazy stuff. Not now while I'm tryin' to relax and be a positive person. I want to change my life around, which is truthfully and sincerely what I've been tryin' to do."

Mark paused, lost in thought. "You know?"

Mark sat forward and wrapped his hands around his injured thigh. "This thing hurts," he said, rubbing it gently. He pulled off the brace and showed me the wound. The scar was long, running most of the way down his thigh. It was clean, and the staples looked secure. He ran his fingers along it and grimaced as he pressed each staple.

"It's going to be sensitive when you press on it," I told him. "There's a lot of swelling and the nerves are damaged too. But it looks like it's healing well, and I don't see anything that looks like an infection."

Mark sighed. "That makes me feel better, 'cause they were talking about how it could get infected," he said. "I don't got no more pain medication, and I have a lot of pain."

"Why haven't you called your doctors?" I asked him.

"'Cause the doctors were treatin' me like shit. I mean, they wasn't treatin' me good at all, man. Nurses wasn't comin'. I called 'em, but they didn't come. I think my medical care wasn't right, man. So I'm stickin' it out and tryin' to get better. But, like I keep sayin', till I met you, my medical care was shitty."

I thought back to six weeks before, when I met Mark in the hospital. I went by late one morning and found him in a double room. He didn't wait for me to introduce myself before letting me know how unhappy he was with the medical care he was getting. In his rhythmic, husky voice, he explained, "I got shot in the leg. Doctors had to bypass the artery in this leg. They told me they almost had to amputate my leg. But when I ask for pain medication, the nurses just tell me 'tolerate it.' I just feel like gettin' up out of here. Why should I stay if they're not gonna help me?"

Because of Mark's distress, I made a call to Cil, the head nurse on the unit, to see if she could talk with him about what his troubles were. When I saw Mark the next day, he seemed better and gave me credit (more than I deserved) for the intervention of the head nurse. He told me how bored he was and that he had no money to have the television turned on. I gave him a few dollars for the television, and his initial suspicion of me seemed to fade quickly. I came back to see him several times, and Mark seemed pleased to have someone coming by to check on him.

There was a long weekend, after which I came back and found that he had been discharged. I saw him when he returned for a follow-up appointment in the surgical clinic. But then he disappeared to New Jersey to stay with his mother. He left me his phone number there, and I talked to him several times. He seemed content, but later, he told me that his mother's drug use was becoming a problem and that she was difficult to live with. He complained a lot about his pain and how he hadn't been seen by the doctor and how he didn't even have an appointment scheduled.

So, when he came back into town, I had him come to the hospital to see me in the clinic. There, the nurse helped clean up his wound, and the clinic psychologist talked to him about the trauma he had been through. Afterward, we connected him with the social worker, who helped him fill out social security disability forms. These few things seemed routine to us, but to him, they seemed to contrast with his days on the acute surgical unit. Still, his resentment over that time had not yet eased.

■ ■ ■

Now, listening to Mark in his apartment, his voice grew singsong and strident as he listed out his complaints about his care. "I even wrote a letter about it, about my medical care."

"Did you?" I asked. "Who'd you send that to?"

"I didn't send it to anyone. But I wrote about things that was goin' on. Waitin' forty-five minutes to take painkillers and stuff like that when I was really hurt.

"I'm messed up in my head now too. I keep seeing their faces, whoever shot me. Just going through mad scary feelings right now, and just tryin' to be strong. But I just keep seeing that day in my head."

Mark flopped back onto the bed like he was weary of perching himself on his elbows. "The road to recovery's been hard! Just livin' day by day. I'm barely makin' it. Barely makin' it. Barely makin' it."

"What do you mean?"

"I'm just livin' right by the skin of my teeth now. My father brings me one meal a day. I don't have no source of income. I have two little boys that I really love and usually take care of them. But for the last month and a half almost, since I got shot, I haven't been able to do anything for them. So, you know, mentally, I'm pretty messed up. Physically, I'm pretty messed up. But I'm really tryin' to work to get better.

"I gotta go to the bathroom," Mark said suddenly. He gathered his crutches, pulled himself up and steadied himself for a moment before easing out of the bedroom and through the now-dark kitchen. I suddenly realized that I had been there for more than an hour. The bright summer light had faded into twilight, and the streetlights were on. The poorly lit apartment was growing dim, and for the first time, I began to feel nervous. Mark had already told me he didn't feel safe here. I lived not far away, in Roxbury, which was not much different from Dorchester, a neighborhood many of my friends and colleagues considered too dicey to visit. But my home, at that moment, felt a world away. It was hard to bear the thought of this slight young man alone up here, even with his tough-guy history and exterior.

Mark returned from the bathroom and lowered himself onto the bed. He looked up at me, half-smiling, and said, "You're making me depressed."

"We really don't have to talk about this anymore if this makes you feel bad," I said apologetically.

Mark brightened quickly and smiled, "No, I am just kidding."

With this joking admission, I felt more reluctant to leave. "I am worried about you up here by yourself. You told me you don't feel safe here. What can I do that would help you?"

"Don't worry, Doc," he said, "I've been livin' out on my own ever since I was fifteen. Livin' in the streets, livin' in cars. Takin' showers outside with water jugs. Buyin' new socks every day, new soap every day. I used to literally go in bushes where no one could see me and take off all my clothes in the bushes, out in the streets, pourin' water on me, washin' my body. I had a rough life, man. I had to learn the hard way. This is nothin' compared to that.

"I do think about whoever shot me, though. Like, are they gonna try and come in my house or shoot my windows out or somethin', you know? I think maybe while I'm layin' in bed, you know, someone might climb up on my porch and shoot through the window. I just think about things like that. You know?"

Mark leaned forward. "But let me tell you how I've been raised by my grandmother: to be strong. She was a church lady, but she said, 'If people mess with you, there's always a stick, a brick, or bottle or somethin'. Or if not, then run.'" He chuckled. "She always told me that, so I know how to fight."

"You said your father comes by to help you out, right?"

"Yeah he helps me out. He's really all I got 'cause my mom is messed up off drugs. She was locked up too. I didn't even meet her until like I was ten or eleven. But, she still drinks, so she got her own problems. Right now, I'm just in this world by myself.

"That's why I'm tryna cut down on smokin' weed. I've seen what all those drugs have done to my family. I ain't smoked weed since . . . let me see. I ain't smoked it since I was in the hospital."

"While you were in the hospital? When you went downstairs or something?" I asked.

Mark laughed. "Yeah, one time. My friend came and pushed me all the way around the corner, to like the next street over? You know that little alley?" He chuckled again.

"I went right back in the hospital. Just relaxed and laid down. Had a good day. Got my appetite back. 'Cause before that, I wasn't eatin' anything. I couldn't shit. Nothin'. Once I took a toke of that weed, I went and ate some food, and the next mornin', took a shit! It was hard, like a *rock*! Really, it was petrified stone!"

Mark shrugged. "I don't know why I smoke weed. I guess from smokin' weed for so long. It's just a habit."

We both left space for a long pause, and Mark reached over and gathered one of the charcoal-colored cats that was rubbing itself on his brace and pulled it onto his lap.

"Really, I can just keep on talkin' about my life, you know? You can ask me any question and I'll tell you the truth. That's one thing I do.

"Like, I might lie to get outta trouble. But I don't lie to make a conversation. You feel me? Now, some people, they just lie just for anything. That's stupid."

He looked up at me. "I seem like I've answered those questions pretty honestly, right?"

"Absolutely," I answered. "I appreciate that. And I hope we will get the chance to talk again."

I motioned toward the stereo on the floor. "On my way out, do you want to let me hear one of your rhymes?"

"Oh, all right. We can do that," Mark said, looking pleased to be asked. He slid to his right and hit the play button on the stereo. The speakers pumped out a dense beat, and Mark's head began to bounce. "This is somethin' Boston, a little somethin' I try and take care to be positive. So, check it out."

Like a performer on stage, Mark's voice now deepened and grew louder. "My agenda each day was pumpin' coke, twenties and dimes and nickles I sold for smoke. . . ." he sang out. Among images of dope fiends complimenting the quality of his crack cocaine and "bitches" who hung on his every move, Mark described the lucrative and dangerous business of bagging up drugs to "pump out on the Boston streets."

Mark let the beat fade out, looking proud of the rhymes he had delivered. I nodded and said, "Good," all the while aware of the disconnect between his stated desire to be positive and the drug-laced rhyme that he had so effortlessly produced.

Mark popped up and grabbed his crutches. We walked to the door, and he removed the flimsy barricades.

"You don't have to come down with me," I told him.

"Yeah, I do," he corrected me. "I gotta lock the door."

I walked down, and he followed me, taking one step at a time until I was delivered again to the entrance. "Thanks again for all you did for me," Mark said. I nodded and shook his hand. He pulled my arm and leaned his shoulder into my chest in that way that black men hug each other. He hobbled inside, and I heard the door bolt.

I walked out into the damp summer evening, and the black dog charged me again. I strode deliberately through the yard to my car. A few people were out in the summer evening air. Men and women and children were sitting on their porches across the street. We nodded to each other but did not speak. I got into my car and drove the short distance to my house.

10

KARI IN HIS GRANDMOTHER'S HOUSE

Six weeks after Kari and I sat together in the surgical clinic, I drove to Hyde Park to meet him at his grandmother's house. The house sat on a narrow two-way street not far off American Legion Highway, which lies just off Blue Hill Avenue, the main road that cuts through Roxbury, Dorchester, and finally Mattapan before coursing out of the city into the suburb of Milton. The house sat midway down a long row of attached two-story houses, a noticeable contrast from the century-old triple-deckers that lined Blue Hill Avenue standing directly opposite these more modern and modest homes.

Kari met me at the door and motioned me to come inside, taking a moment to scan the street before following me inside. The Venetian blinds were drawn closed, and the small living room felt close and dark. The furniture was vintage 1970s, the upholstered gold chairs draped in thick plastic. The carpet seemed to me to be the same grass-green pile rug that I had grown up with. Perched on faux-marble end tables were fading black-and-whites of a gleeful young woman being held by a mustached man with his hair slicked back.

Kari invited me into the small square kitchen, where I took

the seat at the table across from him. It was after 5 p.m., and the late autumn light outside was starting to fade. A small lamp mounted above the table glowed with our only light. The kitchen was tidy, and the clean appliances, though also more than 20 years old, sparkled like new. The counters held ceramic canisters painted to look like miniature bungalows. The kitchen table was white Formica with specks of gold, and the table top was wrapped with a thick metal band decorated with wide ridges. It reminded me of the table in my grandmother's kitchen.

Kari slumped in his chair. He had lost weight. There was an air of sadness about him. He looked down much of the time and smiled less than before, rarely flashing his brilliant white teeth.

"What has life been like for you?" I asked.

"Well, they caught the dude that shot me. That's one good thing. They told me that he just got out of court that same day for armed robbery." He sighed heavily. "That's the crazy part. They was all set to send him away, but they let him out 'cause his mother's disabled. They say she needed him to take care of her. So, they let him go and he comes and shoots me."

"I never even seen that dude before. Or maybe I seen him once. Now I can't get this dude out of my head. I see him every day, every night, even though he's locked up. And now I have to deal with what people on the streets are sayin'."

"Like what?" I asked.

"That I snitched on him and stuff like that. But I don't let that bother me. But that's the word on the street, I guess."

"Why are they saying that?"

"Because I told the cops that he did it. But I feel like he put *himself* there. He threw the gun right down the street from where he shot me. I didn't turn him in. He did it to himself."

"So, what do they think you should have done?"

"I don't know. I guess they think I shoulda tried to handle it myself. But that's crazy. That's how people go to jail." He scratched at an area of dried skin on his hand and looked nonchalant.

"I used to care what other people thought before I got shot. Now I don't care what people think about me. I'm still livin'. So hey, they can say whatever they want. They ain't feedin' me. They ain't puttin' no clothes on my back. They ain't givin' me a place to live. They can say whatever."

"How about physically? Do you feel like you're getting better?" I asked.

"Yeah, probably, but I don't really know. I hope I don't be hunched over forever. I don't know why the doctors cut me up like this, man. I got shot in the back, but they cut me in my stomach. I don't understand why they cut me in my stomach. They cut me from here, all the way up to like right here, but I got shot over here."

Kari lifted his shirt to show me where the bullet entered, but my eyes were immediately drawn to the scar that ran down his belly. The mark stood out against Kari's smooth onyx skin. It was deep and not completely straight. Starting just below his ribcage, it ran down the middle of his abdomen, looped around his navel and disappeared beneath his jeans. The scar was flanked on either side by rows of protruding, scarred flesh. The wide scar cut through his young body the way a plow cuts through soft earth, leaving mounds of soil along its furrow. These sides were not smooth but were interrupted every 3 inches or so by a band—remnants of stitches—that bunched the troubled flesh into rough bulging segments. I recognized this appearance as a sign that the surgeon was forced to let the wound heal on its own, from the bottom up—"secondary intention," it was called—as a way to prevent a serious infection.

"They said the bullet's still in my chest. And now I'm scared about that, because they're talkin' about if it ever moves, I have to come back to the hospital to get operated on, and they gotta put the chest tubes back in. And I don't think I can take that again. My ribs are still sore from those chest tubes.

"So, I ain't goin' through that again. I just can't. Unh-unh." Kari shook his head, clearly dreading the thought.

He paused. "In a way I blame myself for it. I should have just given him my chain. That way, I could have avoided all this. I almost lost my life over it. I don't even wear a chain no more. I got a gold watch too. I don't even wear that. I wear this cheap one instead." Kari stretched out his arm and turned his wrist back and forth. The watch was a Timex, the kind of watch they sell at Walgreens and CVS.

"I was innocent, and I got shot. So, anything can happen. Anything. Everybody kept tellin' me that life is like that. Anything can happen."

"Have you been concerned about your safety?" I asked.

"Yeah, sometimes. I don't wanna walk past where I got shot. I'll never go up that way no more. But I don't even let that get to me.

"I just think, if I was to get in that predicament now, I wouldn't try to push him, I would just give it to him. It ain't worth it. I'm not even gonna get another chain. It ain't even worth it no more."

"What are you thinking about for the future?" I asked.

Kari smiled for the first time. "I think about the future a lot. I always wanted to be a model, you know?"

"A model?" I asked.

"Yeah, man. I always wanted to be a model like that dude 'Tyson. I wanted to, but after I got shot, it messed up my body. Now I got scars and stuff.

"I wanted to do a lot of things. I shoulda just went to school, like everybody was tellin' me to." His smile faded into regret.

"What do you think you'll be doing in five years?" I continued.

"In five years? I know what I'm gonna be doin'. I'm gonna be in A&R."

"What's that?" I asked.

"Artists and Repertoire. Like findin' young talent? 'Cause my friends just signed a record deal. And they'll get like a $80,000 advance. So, they was gonna buy a three-family house and turn it into their own studio. I was gonna be their A&R, findin' the groups, gettin' 'em in the studio, makin' sure they do what they gotta do. 'Cause they gonna open up their own record label, eventually. That's my plan. That's an option."

I remembered now Kari's friend Marlon, who weeks ago looked so proud when he talked about his successful contract. Now there was an uncertainty in Kari's voice that made me wonder if this dream would become a reality.

"Everybody's tellin' me to go to college, but I don't think I'm a college-type person. I probably could go, but that don't fit me. Not a college boy.

"I barely got outta high school. Barely, but I made it out. I wasn't doin' my work. I was chasin' after girls. But that's the environment I was in. I don't think I could handle college life. I'd be goin' crazy from all the stress, man. I hate stress.

"It's for the better, I think. I wasn't like the perfect kid, but I wasn't a bad kid. But now, I'm a good kid. That's how I look at it now. I ain't a man just yet, but I'm soon to be. I want to live to see myself be a man and my son to be a man."

These words came out earnestly, as if Kari wanted to believe them, even if he could not, entirely. He looked straight at me now and a dullness inhabited his eyes. The optimism of months before was fading, overtaken by regret. I thought back to several months ago, when Kari told me that getting shot was his "wake-up call." But now it seemed that that window of opportunity for Kari to see his injury as an act of grace from God had begun to close. It was as if he were trying to catch up to where he was in the week or so after he had gotten shot. In the months that had passed, the daily tasks of trying to recover his strength while also acting on his promises to change his life had worn him down and left him adrift.

I recognized something in Kari that I had seen in other young patients who had suffered near-fatal trauma. In the days and weeks after the injury, the transient light of hope and possibility burns remarkably bright. Even then, it can be hard to detect this hope in their numbed, expressionless faces. But it came through loud and clear in their words.

But if this small fire lit by the near-death experience was not kindled, often it was smothered by the burdens that began to accumulate in their lives. Families and friends grew tired of the routine of caring for young men who should, in their estimation, have reverted to the vibrant teenagers they had been just months before. Regrets, disfigurement, pain, and fear rolled together and blurred their hopes for the future.

"But you know I'm not giving up, Doc," Kari said, interrupting my thoughts as if he had heard them. "I know I'm gonna be all right. I gotta be all right, gotta make it for my son."

"I hear you," I told him. "And I agree. You need time to heal."

Kari nodded as he pushed himself up from the chair with a faint grunt and walked me through the living room and toward the front door.

When I left Kari, it was dark. Still, as I walked to my car, I strained to see the spot where Kari had fallen and the place where he later had lain in the street, wondering whether he would live or die. But there was nothing that marked this place for me. Because Kari was alive, there was no shrine of teddy bears, Botanica candles, or half-sipped bottles of Hennessy marking the place where he might have taken his last breath. The exact spot, though, was precisely etched in Kari's memory and his aching, scarred body.

I made my way back down American Legion Highway, along the edge of Franklin Park and onto Blue Hill Avenue, retracing the route that the ambulance carrying Kari likely took. Not many people were moving in and out of the humble storefronts of bodegas, hair salons, and liquor stores that lined this main drag. The air had taken on a decided chill, and Bostonians were not yet acclimated to the coming winter.

11

JIMMY IN JAIL

One warm afternoon in late spring, I found myself driving up Route 2. It was a long drive, but once I left Boston, the scenery became green and lush. The highway was flanked by verdant forest interspersed with country meadows. The road wound up through the historic town of Lexington and ran lazily toward Walden Pond. As I approached MCI-Concord, I realized how large and imposing it was. So large was it that the road was forced to veer around it.

I pulled off the highway and followed the signs to the main entrance. I passed a large granite marker that announced the prison and displayed the names of the governor and the state's secretary of corrections. Another, smaller sign spelled out a warning that this was a correctional facility, and anyone who was found to be in violation of the law was subject to arrest. These signs made me nervous, not because I had done anything wrong—I had never even gotten a speeding ticket—but because I was a black man, I always grew a bit tense. I imagined myself a character in some Hollywood nightmare thriller where I knew that I was a doctor but all the world believed that I belonged behind the prison walls. It was an irrational fear—

and I felt silly for entertaining it. But inside, there was an odd feeling that made me wonder exactly how I would prove, in the event of a bizarre mixup, that I was not one of the black men who had been assigned there.

I drove down the long straight drive, which eventually delivered me to a sprawling new red-brick compound bearing a huge sign that said "Massachusetts Correctional Institution– Concord." I parked in the asphalt lot and walked between the columns of blue Crown Victorias and sheriff's vehicles to the plate glass doors. I stepped inside the sparkling lobby, which looked like it belonged in a building in the financial district downtown. A woman in uniform sat behind the shiny oval orbit disk of a desk in front of a flatscreen computer monitor. She greeted me without smiling, and when I gave her Jimmy's name, she asked for my photo ID. She tapped on the computer keys in front of her and then frowned with a sigh. "He's not here," she said. "This is Concord Maximum. He's in Concord Medium. You have to go back out, make a right out the lot and follow the road all the way. You'll come to it." She recited this from rote, as if she said it many times in the course of a day.

I left the slick-looking Correctional Center and walked back to my car. Sitting in the sun for just 10 minutes, it was no longer cool and airy but stifling. I pulled out of the lot and onto the small access road that led around the back of the maximum-security building and dipped down onto a smaller road that cut along a large pasture. The pasture was green and easy and unoccupied by livestock or any vegetation but grass. It would have been easy to forget for a moment that behind the walls lived hundreds of prisoners who were being held for crimes like murder, rape, robbery, and sexual assault. But the road was lined with tall fences topped by spirals of razor wire. I followed the fences, and after a half-mile I came to a modest complex of prefab-looking buildings set in parallel rows and spread out like bunkers across the wide field. I pulled into the small gravel parking lot. I could only see the first of these low buildings, but even from there, I could sense the expansiveness of the complex.

I gathered up my notebook and pen and entered through the double doors. Inside, a guard sat behind a glass window and gathered forms from the handful of women who had come to visit. A sign on the wall announced that all visitors must complete the visitor's form, so I moved past the line to the counter. The line moved slowly behind me, and in my blue serge jacket and red and blue Hilfiger tie, I felt oddly out of place. I filled out the form, answering "no" to the full list of questions about all the illegal things I might have done in the past or might plan to do during my visit. I walked to the back of the line to wait my turn.

Meanwhile, a young, slender, brown-skinned woman in a blue tank top, a denim skirt, and flip-flops stood at the front of the line, testily answering the guard's questions. Her brown eyes squinted with fatigue and frustration. She held a toddler on her hip, a little girl of perhaps 3 years old who was squirming. She too was wearing flip-flops, one of which had dropped to the floor. The girl arched all the way back so that she was looking at the other people in line upside down and then bounced up with a giggle. When she did this a second time, the distracted mother kicked her hip out to bounce the girl upright and said, "Stop!" Her voice thundered through the empty bunker in a way that made all heads turn. The little girl settled obediently and curled her hand in front of her mouth. Not missing a beat, her mother continued answering the guard's questions with annoyance. No, she was not bringing anything to the inmate. No, she had not been convicted of any felonies.

"I come here every week. Why don't they just write this stuff down?" she asked the other women as she turned to walk to the waiting room. The other women in line said nothing but stayed in line to begin the process themselves.

When I reached the booth, I saw that the officer was an olive-skinned Latino man with thick muscular arms that strained against the sleeves of his blue uniform. He looked over my form and, without looking up at me, asked me to confirm that I understood the rules and that I had not brought anything with me that I intended to give to an inmate.

"What is your relationship to Jimmy Parker?"

I paused for a moment. Then I cleared my throat and said, "I'm a friend."

"A friend?" he asked, looking up at me now for the first time and searching out my eyes.

"Yes. Friend," I said. He flicked up an eyebrow and returned his gaze to the form. He filled out several lines at the bottom of the form, stamped it, and tore off the perforated bottom and handed it to me.

"Where do I go?"

"Just go to the waiting room behind you and wait until they call the inmate's name."

I grabbed the small slip of paper and walked back to an open cinderblock room. The room was filled with black plastic bucket chairs, all of them scarred with scratches and pits. Army-green lockers lined the far wall of the room; to their right was a door in institutional gray. The door was a Dutch door, allowing the top and bottom halves to open separately. I sat down a few yards away from the door, my back to the lockers, and looked out into the room. There were only two other people waiting—a middle-aged African American woman and a young Latina. Both women sat, not looking at me, not looking at each other, not reading a book. They seemed to be in a patient trance, enduring without complaint a process over which they had no control. None of the other women whom I saw in line were still waiting, so I assumed they were already inside. "This must mean that I will not be waiting long," I thought, so I began to flip through my notebook.

After a couple of minutes, I was startled by the loud crack of a bolt being thrown. The upper half of the dense gray door opened, and a tall thin officer with heavily gelled hair called out, "Lopez!" The Latina jumped to her feet and walked quickly to the door, sliding her sandals along the floor with each short step. She handed the officer her piece of paper; after looking it over, the officer closed the upper part of the door and then opened the entire door. The woman disappeared from sight. Another five minutes passed, and the routine with the loud crack and the opening of the door repeated itself, the officer calling "Singletary!" this time. The older black woman passed deliberately through the door, and it slammed shut behind her.

I was left alone in the expansive bunker. I was surprised that there were not more visitors. I had imagined that the place would have been brimming with family and friends, girlfriends and children aching to see their sons, brothers, boyfriends, and fathers.

Twenty minutes passed, and I had not been called. I looked at my watch. It was 2:30. Visiting hours started at 1 o'clock and ended at 4. I realized that I should have expected to wait a long time, but at that point, I was worried about whether Jimmy and I would have any time to talk. Ten more minutes passed, and the door finally opened. The officer leaned out. "Parker!" He shouted it as if I were not the only one sitting in the room. I walked to the window and handed him the small paper, expecting that I would be ushered through the door like the two visitors before me. But the officer stopped me.

"Are you his lawyer?" he asked.

"No," I answered.

"Well then, you can't bring that stuff in here."

I held up the notebook. "You mean this?"

"That, the tie, the jacket. You need to empty your pockets. No phones, no pagers, no money. Take off the belt too. You can put all your stuff in one of those lockers."

"Really?" I asked stupidly.

"That's right. Only lawyers can bring in stuff like that, and you just said you are not his lawyer."

"I'm a doctor," I said, in a lame attempt to defend myself.

"Not in here, you're not," he sniped back with a developing smirk. "Knock on the door when you're done."

I moved to my left and faced the row of lockers. I tried to contain my disgust as I removed all the change and keys from my pockets and slid my pager, cell phone, and watch to the back of the square green box. I slipped off my blazer and loosened my tie to remove it over my head. The space was so small that I had to fold my jacket inside out in order to stuff it into the locker. Finally, I pressed the notebook up against the jacket and held it with one hand while I closed the door with the other. I pressed the door closed and slid two quarters into the slot, which allowed me to remove the plastic orange key.

I went back to the door, knocked twice, and waited for the guard to return. Sitting in the waiting room, I had imagined that on the other side of the door were the small cubicles I had seen on television with a thick slab of bulletproof glass and telephones on either side. But now, stripped down as I was, I could only imagine that there would be no glass curtain. Instead, I envisioned long tables with visitors on one side and inmates on the other, where families could at least hear the clear voices of their loved ones and hold their hands. Perhaps this routine was what made this possible.

After several minutes I knocked again, this time using the side of my hand like a hammer. Within a few seconds the guard opened the entire door, and I walked through into a cramped security room. The guard closed and heavily bolted the door behind us. This was not the visitors' room I was expecting. Another officer was there—a short but thick African American woman with short braided hair and so many implements hanging from her belt that she had to hold her arms out from her body like a gunfighter at a showdown in the Old West. She stood silently as the other guard began to search me.

"You will need to take off your shoes and hand them to me." I obeyed and leaned over to untie my shoes while standing up. I leaned my hand on the wall and pulled off the tight-fitting wingtips. The guard, who by now had donned latex gloves, took the shoes from me and placed them on a table on the other side of a metal detector.

"Now, show me the bottoms of your feet. Turn around. Roll up the collar of your shirt."

I did all of these things, just as he had instructed me.

"Now turn around," he said matter-of-factly. He stepped close to me. "Open your mouth."

"What?"

"I need to look in your mouth to make sure you are not carrying any contraband."

I leaned back away from him and opened my mouth.

"Lift up your tongue." I obeyed, and he peered down into my mouth. "Now lower your tongue." He crouched and leaned in toward my chest so that he could see the roof of my mouth. The strands of hair on his head were gelled together in neat parallel rows, like a freshly plowed field. He was close enough to me that the stale smell of his cigarette breath melded with the unsmoked tobacco in his breast pocket, hitting my nostrils at the same moment. The combination left me nauseated and annoyed. He continued his pro forma examination.

"Now, I want you to walk through this metal detector."

I passed through the chrome and black plastic arch, and it did not make a sound.

"You are all set, then," he told me from the other side of the arch. He pointed to the table next to me where he had placed my shoes. I leaned against the table and slid on my shoes. I fixed the collar of my shirt and stood up, waiting for the next instruction.

Across the small room, the two guards were deep in conversation. They ignored me, as if in the minute that had passed, they had forgotten that I was there. I waited another minute before speaking up. "What do I do now?"

The woman turned and looked at me as if surprised that I was still there. "Oh, honey," she said sounding like someone's mother, "You have to speak up, 'cause we just get goin' and forget about the whole world." She chuckled. "C'mon this way," she said, waving me with her hand. She led me through a large door that opened outside into the bright sun and onto a ramp that forked between two nearby buildings. One ramp led straight ahead into a twin cinderblock building and the other led off to the right, toward a path that wound between the structures. She turned to the right, and I followed. After several steps, she turned and looked back at me sternly.

"Not this way. You go over there," she said, pointing to the other cinderblock building.

I shrugged and explained, "This is my first time here."

"Well, that's the visiting area. This way is restricted." She stood, hands on hips, and watched me retrace my steps to the proper path before she turned and marched off.

In the industrial building, I walked into a small hallway that led to a sprawling room about half the size of a banquet ballroom. A sign announced, "All activities in this room are monitored by security cameras." Across the ceiling at regular intervals, smoky charcoal-colored domes confirmed the presence of video cameras. The floor was gray speckled linoleum, and the ceiling hung low, like storm clouds. There were rows and rows of institutional black plastic chairs that stretched in parallel rows across the width of the room. The chairs were arranged back to back with six feet or so separating the rows. Unlike the waiting room, this space was filled with people, and the air was humid and stale.

Silver-uniformed guards sat at a pentagon-shaped guard station that was set up on a platform elevated a foot or so off the ground. Behind the desk, several guards attended to television monitors, talked into walkie-talkies mounted on the shoulders of their uniforms, and scanned the visitors and inmates in the room.

At the back of the room was a bank of fully stocked vending machines. Visitors, most of them women of various ages and ethnicities, bounced from machine to machine, inserting white plastic cash cards. They looked up and down the contents—Snickers bars, oatmeal creme cookie sandwiches, Slim Jims, potato chips, peanut butter crackers, and all types of soda—and then punched in their selections on the keypads. They collected the sweets and snacks that dropped from the coils before moving into a line at another machine.

I walked down the middle aisle and picked a chair halfway

down the row. I sat and waited with nothing to do—no book to make notes in, no phone to make calls. Off to my right, an elderly woman with wrinkled nut-brown skin pressed her palms against the cheeks of a young inmate. I watched as they leaned into each other. She was smiling so hard that her eyes seemed to disappear into small slits. Fully captive in her hands, the young Latino man, whom I took to be her son, melted into a bashful smile. A young woman in a pink dress sat nearby, smiling as she took in the scene.

Across from me, an olive-skinned woman in a pink flower print summer dress waited, alone. She was an attractive young woman who looked to be in her twenties. Her dark brown shoulder-length hair was freshly styled into a soft curl. Her ankles were crossed, and she was shaking one foot rhythmically to nonexistent music. Her pink and white sandals popped against her heels with each shake. She sat patiently; clearly she had been there for a while. Piled on the seat next to her were snacks she had bought from the machine. Candy bars held up a shiny cinnamon roll, next to onion potato chips and Doritos. Chocolate-frosted cupcakes and a bag of peanuts rounded out the neatly arranged gifts.

I looked around at the clock. It was 3:15, and visiting hours were ending in 45 minutes. I saw why all of these friends and relatives had appeared much earlier than I had. They knew from past visits that the process of getting into this ordinary room could consume an entire afternoon. I had dreaded this trip for the muted terror that I felt entering these walls of confinement, but these feelings were different. The oppressive and uncontrollable tedium of the waiting, preceded by the intrusive search, had numbed me. I was frustrated to have come so far, only to be left with just a few minutes with Jimmy—if I saw him at all.

By this time, a thick man with inky tattoos on his hands and a jet-black crew cut had joined the woman with the mountain of treats. She smiled broadly at him, and he hugged her and swung her from side to side, at one point lifting her off the floor. Then they sat down, and he dug through the pile of snacks like a child looking for his favorite. He opened a cellophane package of small chocolate sponge cakes with white filling and fed her a bite before finishing it himself.

I looked over toward the guard station where the officer had turned his attention back to the desk in front of him. I could not help but notice that all of the guards in the room were white, and most of them were men. A lone woman guard, a redhead, stood near the door that the inmates passed through. It was the opposite for the inmates. I looked around the room, and in small huddles were black or brown men paired with black or brown friends or families. There were a few groups of white people scattered here and there, but to my eye, it was less than a quarter of the men there.

Just after 3:25 the door opened again, and seven or eight inmates came through. Near the back, the shortest of the group, was Jimmy. He was wearing a light blue denim shirt and navy chinos. The group left him behind, as each peeled off to the usual spot where family or friends met them. Jimmy walked more tentatively. He squinted and scanned the room for someone he might recognize. He had a look of curious confusion and intrigue on his face. I stood up and raised my hand as he looked in my direction, an action that seemed to catch the attention of the four or five groups of inmates and visitors who were seated near me.

As Jimmy walked toward me, his face bloomed a smile of relief, like a puzzle had been solved in his mind. He was careful not to accelerate his approach but continued toward me with a cool stride.

"Hey" he said. "I couldn't figure out for the life of me who my visitor was. But you said you was gonna come visit me way back. So I forgot when you was comin'." He walked toward me and took my hand and pulled me toward him. We hugged politely while our hands remained interlocked between our chests. He sat down.

"So you made it up here okay?" he asked, making small talk.

"Yeah, it wasn't too bad a drive. I have never been up here before."

"Yeah, it's pretty close, but still far if you ain't got a car. That's why my peoples tell me they don't be comin' up here. No car. . . . Even though they could probably get one if they wanted to, you know what I'm sayin'?

"You 'bout the only person who came up to see me the whole time I was here. No, wait. My mother came up here one time, and she brought my sisters. But that's pretty much it. My lawyer comes up, but that don't count. That's her job."

"What about your father?" I asked.

"He's still locked up. But he should be getting out in a couple of months."

Jimmy sat forward now, changing the subject entirely.

"Did I tell you about the appeal I'm goin' through?"

"Yeah, you did. In your letter. How's that going?"

"I think we got a good chance. My lawyer do too. 'Cause the people that got robbed? They got a totally different description of the dude that did it."

"I'm just 5 feet, 5 inches. They said the guy was like 6 feet— 7 inches taller. And dark-skinned. I'm brown-skinned. So we got a pretty good chance. At least I hope we do. That's what she say."

He twisted his head and put his hand to his chin. "What do you think?" he asked me.

"Hmmm, I'm not a lawyer. I hope your lawyer's right. But even then, these things are hard," I said vaguely.

"Yeah, I guess you're right." He leaned back in the chair, somewhat deflated.

He turned and caught the eye of a thin young black man with a bushy black beard. " 'Sup T," he said. "That your lady?"

"Yeah," the man said, grinning and cocking his head toward the woman. They talked for several turns before Jimmy's deep, harmonica voice caught the attention of a correction officer who looked up from the desk. Jimmy saw this out of the corner of his eye, because he immediately turned back to me.

"The guards. They just be on you all the time. No matter what you do, some of them just be assholes. There's a few that's okay, but most of them just love their jobs too much."

I nodded in sympathy, but I tried to take us back to the topic of the date of his eventual release. I had heard the stories of lawyer appeals before from patients in clinic who languished in jail, waiting for the magical appeal to spring them loose. Jimmy's hopes might be similarly destined to disappoint, but I could not tell.

"Jimmy, when are you supposed to get out? I know your letter said you have three years left—" Jimmy interrupted me.

"Nah, like I told you, my lawyer thinks this thing can happen. Maybe even later this year."

"I hear you, but sometimes these things can be hard. They don't always go smoothly, you know? I just want you to think about something you can do in the meantime."

"What you mean?" he said, frowning suspiciously and pulling away, like I was trying to feed him unfamiliar food.

"Well, let me just encourage you to do some things while you are here and think about some other things you can do once you get out, like getting your education. Or reading." I felt like I was talking too quickly, pushed by the need to say anything helpful before the guards began to herd the visitors out of the room. "I know you have lots of time on your hands, so the best thing you can do is to try to expand your mind. Whatever you can do to grow your mind."

Jimmy did not wait before rolling his eyes. He raised both hands and waved them back and forth like he had had enough. "I ain't reading no more books. I read so many books that I just swore—no more books."

"There are some new books out there that you might . . ."

"No more books," Jimmy said firmly but without sounding angry. "I got my GED in here. Then I read all kinds of books, any book that you got or can name, I read it. I decided then that I ain't reading no more books." He seemed sure that this should be the end of the conversation.

"What if I send you some books?" I said, pressing on against his protests.

"You can't," he said with certainty. "They won't let you. You can't send nothing in here except letters and money orders to use in the canteen."

Jimmy turned and looked over his shoulder at the wall clock behind him. "They gonna make me go back in about 15 minutes, but we can stay until they start announcing," Jimmy said, apparently wanting to slow my departure. I looked up at the guard desk where several of the correctional officers were beginning to stand impatiently.

Jimmy's voice softened to a small private tone, as though he was treating me to a secret. "I told you my family don't do nothing for me here. I be up here without a thing. I don't even have deodorant. Not even the cheap stuff they have here." He paused. "Can you help me out with that?"

Having now planted his chair firmly on its four legs, Jimmy waited for my answer, having now turned the conversation back on me. I could not blame him for thinking to ask. Without any visitors and in such distant isolation, who else could he ask? I did not take this personally, but I felt put on the spot. "I'll see, man," I said, hedging. "I'll try to do something for you."

"If you could, Doc, I would really appreciate it." Jimmy was sincere in this, I was convinced, and I resolved to send him something. "One more thing," he said, having extracted what sounded like a promise. "There's this girl I been talking to in New Bedford, and she wants to come up here to see me. But she doesn't know how to get here. She has no idea."

"Yeah?" I asked, unsure if he was about to ask me to drive the two hours down to the troubled seaport city on Cape Cod to pick up a girl and drive her to him.

"Since you know how to get up here, could you write down the directions how you got here and send it to her?"

"Sure, I can do that. But if she has a computer, she can just go to MapQuest and get the exact directions from her house."

"That's the thing," Jimmy said. "She don't have a computer like that."

"Okay then, I can print it out and send it to her. Do you know her address?"

Jimmy twisted his mouth with frustration, eager to solve this before I left. "I gotta get it from her. Sometimes she stays with her grandmother." He stopped again to think. "You could send it to me. Then I can send it to her." He beamed with satisfaction.

"Fine. I will try to do that this week. But, do one thing for me."

"What?"

"When you get out—and I know that might not be for a while—but when you do, I want you to hook up with someone I know who can help you stay straight."

"Who's that?" he said with some suspicion.

"A guy named Roy. He's been through a lot of stuff too, and he's doing pretty well now. He works in a senator's office and he knows a lot about getting back on track and taking care of your kids. He was locked up for a couple of years, but now he is doing really well."

"Yeah," he said with a serious look. "I could do that. I need somebody like that."

"Good," I said, feeling suddenly as if this single pledge had made the journey worthwhile.

By then, the other inmates were starting to peel themselves reluctantly away from their ambivalent families and clinging girlfriends and trail back toward the door through which they had entered. Jimmy looked around and nodded again at his buddy, who watched us closely as he eased down the aisle dragging his untied Nikes with every step.

A minute later, a corrections officer's voice boomed over the loudspeaker: "Visiting hours are over. All inmates gather at the front of the room. All visitors must remain in their seats until you are cleared to leave."

Jimmy stood and grabbed my hand to shake it. "Thanks for

coming all the way up here. That made my day. Only next time you should come earlier." He chuckled.

I nodded, but this time, I made no promises. Instead, I eased to another subject. "Let me know how things go with your lawyer, okay?"

"I will," Jimmy promised as he began to walk away back toward the door. "Keep your fingers crossed."

I watched Jimmy walk away from me, his wide frame holding up the saggy pants and his chubby, still-childlike strut easing back into a protective glide as he rejoined his people. He merged into the small crowd of inmates, each of whom was being checked by a pair of guards. After they confirmed that each inmate was who he was supposed to be, another guard opened the steel door, and each man casually disappeared behind it.

A short, wide officer in a navy uniform and black boots walked up and down the rows of visitors, looking each of us closely in the face to make sure that no inmates remained among us. He looked very young and not menacing at all. But he carried a large black gun on his hip, and as he passed, I could see the crosshatched waffle pattern on the handle closer than I had ever seen it. I felt my heart quicken.

All of us who were visitors continued to sit captive to the prison, restrained in our melamine bucket chairs without permission to rise or to leave. I did not have any sense what the penalty would be for attempting to leave or whether I had the prerogative to inform the guards that I was late and had to get back to my office. But judging from the resignation and patience of the people who were waiting along with me, I could only assume that they had already tried any ideas that I might have and had failed. I was not interested in testing this myself.

Her man now gone, the plump woman across from me folded her hands across her belly. She tapped her foot more slowly than before, looking perfectly content to stay put. I imagined that she had no interest in crossing the guards or risking being barred from her regular visits. Looking warm and satisfied as she did, I knew that she would be back sometime soon to begin her routine of preparing the mountain of snacks and engaging with her ever-widening lover, who would lift her up again.

I, on the other hand, knew that I would not be back. I felt bad, hearing in my head Jimmy's advice about coming earlier next time. But the process of entering, and now leaving, made me numb and anxious. I would see Jimmy when he emerged from prison and returned again to his Dorchester neighborhood. My mission—though I could not have articulated it when I had arrived—was done. Jimmy would connect with Roy, and this, I was sure, would help him.

Finally, a tall guard with a small, tidy mustache strode to the desk and lifted the microphone. "Visitors may exit through the same door through which you entered," he announced before muting the microphone with an electronic squeal. The crowd rose as if a choir director had invited us to stand, and we all moved in a mass to the door.

I wanted to move faster than the shuffling pace and dart through the families to the door, but I feared that any unusual activity might actually slow my exit from the low hanger of a building. So I stayed with the crowd of black and brown people with whom I had coalesced. We inched toward the bottleneck at the door, where yet another corrections officer surveyed our faces for fugitives. I saw the blank faces around me. Most looked calm and routine rather than anxious. I listened to the murmuring of the mothers and wives and girlfriends. The elderly Latina rested her coarse cheek against her daughter's shoulder as they glided, dreamlike, to the exit. I was still impatient, but for most of the people around me, this was a solemn ritual of finding again the men that they had lost. At first it was like they were strolling out of the gates of a cemetery, having meditated on the cold grey granite of a grave marker. Only these were no slabs of stone but living, breathing, fatter and more muscular sons, husbands, fathers, and boyfriends. They seemed grateful these men were safe and sober behind these walls. They had found these men alive, even if in this awful place. Each man could be quickly located with a phone call or a letter. And the hour-long drive up lush green Route 2 could bring loved ones to his side.

I drank all this in as we slowly approached our last checkpoint, where a final guard, this time a beefy redheaded woman with fierce eyes, would certify that we were the same ones who had come in and then sweep us out with a casual wave of her hand. In what seemed like just a moment, I was standing at the door of my steaming green Acura and, in another, was coursing down the emerald green highway toward the city, unsure if I would ever make this drive again.

■ ■ ■

A few days later, I did the two things I promised Jimmy I would do. I stopped by the post office and bought a $25 money order. I printed his name on it and slipped it into a plain white envelope.

Then I sat down at my computer and mapped out directions from New Bedford, Mass., to Concord, Mass. I printed out the paper with turn-by-turn directions and a brightly colored map that plotted out a drive of over 95 miles in blue and yellow. On a 3-inch Post-it note, I penned the words "Jimmy, here are the directions for your friend. I hope it helps." I stuck this to the sheet of directions and tucked it into the same white envelope. With uncharacteristic focus and purpose, I stamped and mailed it the same day. I hoped that the act of helping Jimmy have another visitor would ease my guilt over not repeating the visit myself.

Less than a week later, in the early evening, I was sitting at home in the oversized beige chair that usually lulled me to doze after a fatiguing day of work. The phone rang and the caller ID read "MA Department of Corrections." I answered to a recording that announced, "This call is coming from an inmate at a correctional facility. If you choose to accept this call, you will be charged for the cost. This call is subject to monitoring by law enforcement personnel. If you do not want to accept this call, please press 2. If you would like to accept this call, please press 1."

I pressed "1," certain that I had been charged for the 20 seconds consumed by the wordy warning. In a few seconds, Jimmy's familiar voice confirmed that he was the caller.

"Hey, Doc."

"Hi, Jimmy."

"Thanks for taking my call. I'll try not to talk too long."

"Don't worry about it," I said. "Did you get the stuff I sent you?"

"Oh man," Jimmy said lifting his voice in frustration. "That almost got me in a lot of trouble!"

"How?" I asked dumbly, realizing instantaneously how naive I had been.

"Yeah, the COs called me in the office, 'cause they thought I was tryna plan some kind of escape. They yanked some of my privileges over that, but they know I wasn't tryna do nothin'. Why would I do that? My lawyer's gonna get me out of here with this appeal."

Jimmy said something else, but I was distracted by the thought that I had sent a detailed map to an inmate in a high-security state penitentiary. How could I have done this so absentmindedly? I wondered briefly whether Jimmy could have duped me, playing on my naivete to feed a real scheme. I thought back to how he had flipped my offer to send him books into a request for cash. I could hear him telling me that there was no way to send the directions to his girlfriend but that I should send them to him instead. These thoughts made me interrupt whatever Jimmy was saying. "Jimmy, didn't you know that if I sent you a map, you might get in trouble? I mean, isn't that one of the rules there?"

"Nah, Doc," he protested loudly, "I wasn't even thinking like that. Nobody never sends me nothin'. How could I know that?"

"Okay," I said, not completely satisfied.

"But I really appreciate the money you sent me. Now I got deodorant. I ain't funky no more." He laughed, and I smiled, but barely. Jimmy sensed and filled the brief silence. "Well, Doc, I don't want to run up your bill, but I just wanted to say thanks for you comin' up to see me and for the money. I won't forget it."

"I just want to see you do well when you get out of there," I said.

"I will," Jimmy said. "You watch."

I hung up and flopped back into the chair, which sagged with the imprint of my back and legs. I laughed out loud, thinking that I had been so simple as to send a map to an inmate in a high-security prison. No doubt, my name had already made its way onto a list of suspicious visitors and felons who would be turned away on any future visits. I could see a computer emitting a beep and correction officers raising their heads to talk to each other in low tones if I ever walked in the door. My jail paranoia went no further than this as I drifted off into sleep, thoroughly convinced that they would never have the chance. I could not wait to see the look on Roy's face when he heard what I had done.

12

ROY IN THE PIZZERIA

Sometime in the next fall, Roy disappeared. Roy had been working in Senator Kerry's office on a yearlong internship. The year was drawing to an end, and as expected, he was the darling of the office. Everyone seemed to have adopted Roy and his hard-edged ways, and they were beginning to talk about giving him a full-time job in the senator's office. I remember hearing that Roy had been at the office's annual picnic and softball game that was held on the Esplanade, the park that runs along Charles River. According to a co-worker of Roy's, Roy had ridden his bike and brought his trademark backpack, but more ominously, he had worn a black hooded sweatshirt even though it was the middle of the summer. Roy even got a hit each time he stepped to the plate, 4 for 4, three home runs. But when the game was over and Roy climbed on his bike and headed back toward Roxbury, that was the last they saw of him.

I tried many different ways to reach Roy, paging him multiple times a week over the next few months, but he never called back. He stopped showing up at the CLUB meetings, and because I was unsure precisely where he was staying, I didn't try to look for him. It became clear that, for one reason or another, Roy didn't want to be found.

I remembered his cryptic references about how things were still "hot" in his neighborhood. I didn't know exactly what that meant or what role it might have played in his disappearance. I would have been incredibly worried if Edwin, one of the mentors in the program, had not been there to reassure us. Edwin was a strapping six foot five African American man with haunting green eyes who had spent time in prison; in fact, his time there had briefly overlapped with Roy's. Although he never quite said so, we all believed that he knew where Roy was. He reassured us, without being specific, that Roy was all right but that he couldn't surface.

This too seemed strange to me. Since Boston was such a small place, it wasn't clear to me how Roy could just vanish. There were only so many places that one could go or, I should say, avoid. Places like Downtown Crossing, Dudley Square, the Stop & Shop on American Legion Highway—all were the places that Roy frequented, so I expected that I might run into him at some point. But something else was at work that I didn't understand. I was certain that Roy had not decided to reimmerse himself in the life of crime and drugs that he had disavowed when we were in Washington together. He had been resolute then. He admitted that it was harder to do the good things, like getting up each morning and getting on the train and working long hours to collect a modest paycheck, than it was to live the more profitable life selling drugs. All of that had landed him in jail and had separated him from his family. He had no intention of going back.

Still, I was confused by the way he had disappeared, and I continued trying to make contact with him, futilely paging him, hoping that he would show up or reply—even if only to let us know that he was all right. For the meantime, we had to be content with the assurances of Edwin, who said simply, "Give Roy time. He just has some things to work out."

More than a year later, I dialed Roy's number, as I did peri-
odically on the off chance Roy might call back, and paged him
from the phone in my office. I was working late, and the office
was deserted. I had gotten so used to getting no response to
these pages that I jumped when the phone rang. It was Roy. He
tried to speak as if nothing had happened, as if we had spoken
earlier the same day or several times in the past week.

"Hey, what's up?"

"Roy?" I answered with some relief. "I was worried about
you."

"Yeah, I know. Edwin told me that lots of people have been
asking about me. I'm okay, I guess."

"Where are you?" I asked, probing to see if his call meant
that he was in some dire trouble, thinking he would only call
with a great need.

"I'm all right," Roy said. A long silence hung in the air between us. "You got some time?" he asked. "I need to talk."

"Sure," I told him. "Where can we meet up?"

"Someplace out of the way," he said quietly. I thought ner-
vously about what he meant, what kind of danger he might be
in. Where could we meet that would be safe for him? I remembered a pizza shop in Brookline where a group of us had met
once before. It was far from Roy's neighborhood but close
enough to the T that it would be easy for him to get there if he
did not have a car.

"How about the Uno's in Brookline?" I asked.

"By Commonwealth?" he asked.

"Yeah, right on the Green Line."

"That'll work."

In the few minutes that it took me to gather my things to
leave my office there began a cold and unrelenting rain, of a
kind that seemed to me unique to Boston. Though it was April,
there was a sense that winter had not yet yielded to spring. It did
not take long for the cold and the wet to penetrate my gray wool
coat. The street was as reflective as glass, making it difficult to

see. Large puddles coated the edges of the road and splashed up onto the sidewalk. Still, there were not many cars on the road, so it only took me 20 minutes to reach the Uno's. I parked a long block away, and the rain soaked my coat in the minute or so that it took me to reach the door. Inside, the host asked if he could seat me. "I'm meeting someone here," I told him.

"Feel free to look around, but I don't think anyone's waiting," he said. I strolled through the tables, but the restaurant was mostly empty. We were only a few blocks away from Boston University, and most of the diners looked to be students splurging on beer and thick pan pizza. I took a seat in the corner, at a high bar table with bar stools, and waited for Roy to arrive. An eager waiter circled by several times, apparently with nothing else to do, so empty was the place. I decided to wait for Roy.

After fifteen minutes or so, I started to wonder whether Roy was really going to show. But just then, I noticed a man in a black pea coat with long, thick braids enter the establishment. It had to be Roy, but he looked different. The last time I saw him, his hair had been groomed into an easy fade. But now he had thick, unruly braids hanging off his head like branches from a tree. He held his head down and scanned the restaurant as if making sure it was safe. When he looked in my direction, I lifted my hand and caught his attention. He did not acknowledge me but surveyed the faces in the restaurant for just a few moments more before walking over toward me. I could tell that he did not want me to shout out his name or run over to shake his hand or hug him or tell him how relieved I was to see him. Rather, he walked quietly over to me and slid onto the other stool at the bar table.

"It's been a long time Roy," I said to him. "It's good to see you."

"Yeah man, it has been." He couldn't say another word before the waiter approached us for our orders. "What'll you gentlemen have?" he asked brightly.

"Heineken and a glass of ice," Roy replied without looking up. The waiter turned to me.

"A sparkling water with lime, and bring us the Buffalo wings?" I said, interested in gauging Roy's interest in food.

"Very good," the waiter scurried off.

"What's been happening, man?" I asked, unable to think of any niceties. "Why so out of touch?"

Roy moved his head back and forth with ambivalence. "I just had a lot of drama that I needed to deal with. And I had to deal with it by myself. I couldn't drag anybody else into it with me, especially the senator and all his folks. Stuff was happening that I couldn't tell you about, couldn't tell anyone about. It woulda looked real bad if something had gone down."

"I'm not sure what you mean Roy," I confessed, feeling in some ways like I was owed an explanation.

Roy looked at me straight in the eye. "You really want to know?" he asked, with a "you asked for it" tone in his voice. "The gunplay is back. It's that deep.

"One morning, I was on my way downtown, and I was cutting through the different buildings like all project kids do. Well, this one morning, I opened a door, and I heard a noise. At first, I thought that it was the doorknob hitting the cinderblock wall. You know how, when the chain on a project door is broken, it doesn't close on its own? It just bangs against the wall and makes that funny sound of metal and brick smashing into each other. The sound kind of becomes a part of you.

"But when I looked up at the door, I saw a hole in the door the size of my finger, and the paint peeled back around the hole, like the skin on a baked potato. For a second, it caught me off guard, and I thought, 'Have I seen this hole in the door before?' Usually I remember stuff like that, because all of those holes have stories attached to them. So I reached up and felt it, like how the peeled paint was exposing fresh door metal, and how the hole was really unfamiliar. All this was happening in an instant but like slow-motion.

"When I finally pushed my finger into the hole, it was still warm, and I was like, 'Oh, shit.' I looked up, and I heard 'foom,

foom, foom.' I didn't really hear the sound clearly, but I saw the flame from the gun and heard a muffled 'bang.' I didn't panic or nothing. I'd been here before. I just stepped back into the hallway, and when the shots stopped, I did what most people I know would do; I looked to see who was shooting at me. When I looked, I saw people running away. And these were people I knew.

"So that's when I realized that a lot of old issues that I thought were gone weren't going away just because I got a job."

Roy paused and looked up from the table to survey the room again. Satisfied that no one could overhear us, he dropped his head and continued to pass a packet of sugar back and forth between his fingertips.

"Then one time, I was in the barbershop, and an old enemy walked in just as the barber made his first cut. We had a funny stare down, but he spun and left. I knew he was coming back, and I knew that if I was there when he got back, we would have had to trade shots right there. So I left, half a haircut and all. And I called the barber afterwards, and the dude did come back, too. That's why I grew these braids. I couldn't really sit still for any extended period of time anywhere, so that was the end of my haircuts."

Roy's story explained the thick rows of hair that hung from his head. They matched the way he carried himself, hunched over like an oak that was beginning to fall. Roy's coat threw off the distinct smell of cigar tobacco mingled with marijuana, so familiar to me from my patients, many of whom smoked five or six blunts a day. The circles under Roy's eyes confirmed that he was exhausted.

"I don't know what to say, man. They offered me the permanent job at the senator's office, and I knew I could do it. But I also could tell that they were starting to like me too much. And I was actually starting to like them too much.

"So when I thought about the fact that somebody tried to shoot me on my way to work, I was thinking, 'How far are they willing to go?' Maybe they'll try something when I'm with my kids, or my girl, or my moms. Shit, maybe they'd even try to get me at the place where I work. Who knows?

"That's when I knew I was kinda playing make pretend, or romanced by some wishful thinking. I had a big mess out there that I had to clean up before I could begin to try to be good. My old shit didn't just go away. Boston ain't that type of city, you can't run from drama here. I couldn't let down people like you and people at the CLUB. And I knew my bullshit would splash on y'all at some point if I got caught for something or whatever. And having my name attached to y'all would've made y'all look bad. Y'all ain't shown me nothing but love, so I just decided to drop out of sight until it was all settled."

Roy's cryptic explanations left me more confused, but I decided not to press the issue. "Roy, couldn't we have helped you figure this out?" Even as the words passed my lips, I knew they sounded a bit silly. Roy knew far more about the projects and his own street world than I could ever understand. He knew what he had to do, or at least he thought he knew. Everything Roy had in his head was based on the way he had been raised and the experiences he had had. Even as I sat there, I desperately hoped and wished that somehow I could change his frame of reference. I wondered if by simply plucking him out, if all of his friends and mentors scraped together a few bucks and got him an apartment on the other side of town, would there be any way to free him from this grim responsibility? Or would he view such a development as running away? To me, it seemed that Roy was running toward the problem, eager to confront it head-on, consistent with the way he was raised. Roy was telling me that he could see no other way. But then why the call, and why this meeting?

Just then, the waiter appeared with a tray of drinks and a steaming dish of chicken wings encircling a ramekin of blue cheese dressing and celery sticks. He placed the glass of ice and the second empty beer glass on the table before placing the green Heineken bottle in front of Roy.

"You can take this," Roy told the waiter, holding the empty beer glass up. The waiter obediently grasped it and placed the rest of the items on the table.

"Anything else?" the waiter asked.

"No, we're fine," I answered. He left again and Roy poured the beer over the ice. It cracked as the foam rose up over the edge of the glass.

"So Roy," I asked, "how can I help?"

"I don't know, man," Roy answered. "That's the question. I just need to work some things out. You can tell all my people not to worry about me, but the reason of staying away is not just for me. It's for them too."

"How so?"

"Well, if people are trying to settle old shit with me, then anybody else who is around me could get caught up in the drama. I've done the same things, so I can't complain about the rules now." Roy continued to look around the room. The door opened and a young Asian couple walked in, laughing. Roy looked at them just like he had at every patron in the restaurant. There was a kind of paranoia in him, like a man who was afraid to sit with his back to the door. It was this constant vigilance that began to unnerve me as well. Was he implying that he was staying away from us to keep us from getting caught by a stray bullet?

"Is it really that bad, Roy?" I asked. Again, he chuckled at my naivete.

"Yeah, it is. But it is going to be resolved soon. Know that. I just don't want y'all giving up on me."

"No one is giving up on you. We just want to know what to think."

"You don't have to think nothing or do nothing," he said with a hint of exasperation. "But don't get the idea that I am about to do something crazy. I already told you that I ain't about to do something that would get me lugged back to jail. And I just told you I ain't about to bring shame to you or any of the people who have had my back. Violence ain't the only way to settle things." He stopped there and twirled the ice in the glass of beer.

I was about to open my mouth again, when a fog lifted in my mind. Roy had not come here for me to help him. He had come to help me and all the rest of us who were wringing our hands and paging him endlessly. He was trying to tell us to step back and let him be. I rolled my head back and took a deep breath.

"I need y'all, but just not right now. This thing will lift soon, and I will be cool."

"I hear you, Roy. I really do."

I did not ask any more questions, even though I was desperate to. I realized, though, that Roy did not have any answers, and my questions were only forcing him to make up answers for my benefit. So we just sat and picked at the chicken drumsticks, turning from time to time to look at the basketball game playing on the widescreen television over the bar.

The waiter brought the check, and I promptly slid a $20 bill into the folder and handed it back. Roy and I walked out into the icy mist. We exchanged handshakes and a half-hug before splitting for the walk back to our cars.

"Be safe, Roy," I called to him.

He turned back without breaking stride and called back to me.

"Ain't no other way."

13

ROY BACK IN TOUCH

Almost a year after we sat together at Uno's, Roy reappeared. Unlike his vanishing, he came back into view quietly, almost as if he had never left. I first heard that Roy was back from Tim Argenon, director of the CLUB Program. I ran into Tim one afternoon in Downtown Crossing, just outside of the old Filene's Basement.

He saw me before I saw him, and he startled me when he reached out from a crowd of people and touched me on the shoulder. We had barely exchanged handshakes when he told me excitedly that he had just come from a meeting with Roy.

"You saw Roy?" I asked. "Where?"

"He came by my office. He's ready to take a job at the senator's office."

"Really?" I said, confused and relieved at the same time. "When did Roy resurface?"

Tim laughed. "It was like he fell out of the sky a couple of weeks ago. Started calling, then showed up ready to get right back on the horse."

"And nothing more about whatever he was trying to deal with?"

"Seems like everything he was worried about has blown over. To be honest, I was just so glad to see him, I didn't ask a whole lot of questions. He seems fine to me, though."

"That's great news," I said.

Tim hurried off down Summer Street. I felt a sense of relief, but questions kicked around my head. What had changed to make Roy ready not only to reappear but also to leap into the job at the senator's office? How would he function there, given how distraught he had seemed the last time I saw him? I tried to halt the growing thread of reservations that scrolled across my mind like a ticker tape. The fact was, somehow Roy had emerged intact from the intense personal crisis he had found himself in. Now was not the time to cultivate new doubts about his future. Roy was back, and for now, that was enough.

Several weeks passed before I was able to reach Roy through his pager, even longer for our schedules to allow us to meet up. I was splitting a set of season tickets to the Boston Celtics that year, and since I knew Roy was an avid basketball fan, I invited him to come with me to one of the late-season games. I knew that the game itself would be meaningless, as the Celtics had no chance of reaching the playoffs. But I had learned that none of that really affected the spectacle of the game, since mediocre contests left lots of time for conversation. Roy gladly accepted the offer to join me, and we agreed to meet at the end of the day at the building where he worked.

I rode the train to Government Center and walked the two blocks past the JFK Federal Building to the twelve-story building where the senator's office was located. The modern red-brick building stood angled toward the corner of the street; in front was a petite rock garden with small trees and a few wrought iron benches. I picked a bench that faced the building and sat scanning the lobby through the plate glass doors for a glimpse of Roy. After just a few minutes, the icy metal began to chill me through my trousers, so I stood and strolled lazily along the garden path.

I had just begun to wonder if I had mistaken the time when

I saw Roy's slender figure emerge from the elevator. I strained to see him clearly through the plate glass. When the lobby door swung open, I was shocked at how different Roy looked. He smiled when he saw how transparently my surprise showed on my face.

"Yeah, I know, man. Everybody is buggin' about my hair."

Roy's head no longer carried the thick fuzzy braids. Instead, his hair had been permed straight. It now lay glossy and flat against the top of his head and was pulled back into a neat ponytail.

Even though the look became Roy, it summoned up words and images from my youth. My mother would have called his hairstyle a "conk," because of what she knew of the scalp-scalding, lye-based relaxers of the 1920s, supposedly originated by Cab Calloway. They were intended to give black men hair that resembled that of the white men they entertained. Roy's reason could not have been more different.

"Well, I couldn't wear the braids in the office. And you know about the troubles I had in the barber shop trying to get my hair cut. So I decided not to cut it but get this perm so I can fit into a business office. I checked it out with a couple of people beforehand, not to get their permission, but just to get their ideas. They said it would work, so here I am."

But again, the look suited him. It was stylish and not completely out of step with what might be expected in a workplace. Even if it was a senator's office.

Roy was comfortably dressed in a brown and white shirt, brown tie, and pants to match. He looked thinner than I had remembered him, but aside from the hair, there was another discernible difference. Gone were the hunched posture and defeated facial expression I had seen a year earlier. It was as though he had been relieved of a burden and reentered the world with a new feeling of freedom.

"C'mon up," he said. "Let me show you where I work." I followed Roy through the lobby to the security desk, where a guard carefully scrutinized my driver's license while Roy waited patiently by the elevator. Once the guard cleared me, I rode with Roy to the tenth floor and followed him into the very official-looking suite that bore the emblem of the U.S. Senate. An African American woman seated behind the long reception desk was gathering her things to end the day. Roy introduced her to me as Evelyn and announced that she was the person who really ran the office. She giggled bashfully, evidently thrilled at the teasing.

"No, my job is to make sure that Roy stays in line," she said pointing at him and wagging her finger.

Roy smiled at her sarcastically before motioning me to follow him into a cramped narrow room that held three or four desks positioned in an awkward configuration in order to make them fit. Roy's desk sat at the far end of the room, near the window, and was recognizable by the array of sports photographs that papered the wall above his desk. A thin white man in his twenties sat at his own desk, stacking papers. He looked very young, like an intern newly out of college, making his way into politics. Roy introduced him by saying, ". . . and that's my knucklehead office mate, Ken," almost as though he were introducing a little brother with whom he shared a bedroom. The young man laughed at the familiarity, and it was immediately apparent this was a place where lots of macho banter went on throughout the day.

Roy announced that we were on our way to the Celtics game, quickly imparting to me that as a Lakers fan, his colleague knew virtually nothing about good basketball. Ken responded with a weak jab at the Celtics, the team that Roy had grown up loving. Roy took the bait of the challenge and began to pepper Ken with a string of statistics to say that the Celtics were a better team than the Lakers, even though all of us knew that this year, the Celtics were nursing a losing record.

I could see how quickly Roy had been able to fit back into the office, even though it had been two years since he last worked there. It was clear that they liked having him there and that he served as a kind of reality check. He was a young man whose life was a human manifestation of the social problems that they were idealistically trying to address. His accessibility, combined with his willingness to challenge them, seemed to charge the place with life.

In a matter of minutes, Roy had packed his things into the miniature backpack before saying goodbye to the office and sliding out the door. On the way out, he pointed out the senator's office and spoke of him with a kind of familiar fondness for his willingness to give Roy this chance.

We rode the elevator down and walked the five blocks down Causeway Street to the Fleet Center, the large arena where the Celtics play. Joining the long line of fans filtering through the turnstiles, we took the escalator to the third level and our seats. Along the way, we grabbed a box of Cracker Jack, bought purely out of the superstition that this sticky sweet popcorn would somehow ensure victory for the struggling team.

In the end, the caramel popcorn did not help, and the team fell behind 15 points to the less-than-stellar Atlanta Hawks. Between the play of the game and the intermittent dance routines and foul-shooting contests in the arena, Roy and I talked, but he did not revisit the pains of the previous year. Instead, he focused on how his new position might help him bring new opportunities to his children. "I feel like this is the time to make sure that school is the top thing for them. All of them like school, and all of them like to read, so in a way, I like to think they got some of that from me."

He paused as the crowd noise swelled and overtook his voice. "But I am glad to be back working. I feel like I have had a kind of wake-up call."

"Tell me what you mean by a wake-up call," I prodded.

"Well, all the stuff I told you about, like folks shooting at me in the projects when I was just making my way to work? Well, all that made me realize how much of a mess I left out here. I knew I had to clean it up before it was possible to move on and do good. I was fucking up my ability to be a parent, whether I was willing to admit it or not. If I could have left Boston, I would have done it. But I couldn't take my kids with me, so leaving was just out of the question. So I had to close the book on some old things and just decide not to pick up no new things. So unless somebody forces the issue, I'm out of it, and I'm clean. None of that mess is going to bubble back up. I didn't rat on nobody. I didn't run from nobody. I didn't hurt nobody. And the courts didn't have to make the choice for me; I made the choice.

"I feel like y'all handed me a new lease on life, but back then, I wasn't ready to sign it. Now, I think I'm ready. Maybe now I can do some of the things you were always trying to get me to do and not have my life interrupted or embarrass y'all. I just need to make the kids my focus and keep building on my professional game, you know, build up my resume. But, to be honest, I really don't care what kind of work I do—I'll dig ditches any day—just so long as I can keep my head above water."

14

ROY SETTLES IN

As the summer sun held its place in the sky deep into the evening, people began to gather in the flat open area near the playground at the entrance to Franklin Park. These people came in suits and skirts, carrying shoulder bags and briefcases and cell phones. They milled around in front of the podium that carried the official seal of the Mayor of Boston, which several men in jeans were setting up. This area of the park seldom held such a group of people. Ordinarily, this space served as a walkway for those making their way to the School Boy Stadium or to the golf course. But today all sorts of people continued to gather for a vigil—ministers, probation officers, teachers, public health officials, community workers—to take a visible stand against the rash of violence that was tearing through the predominantly African American communities in Boston.

Soon the mayor arrived with his entourage; the line of official-looking men and women took their places next to him behind the podium. One of the city officials, an elegant African American woman who directed the housing agency, greeted the audience and introduced the mayor. He stepped to the podium and read earnestly from the index cards that held his

speech. He offered words of concern about the violence sweeping through Boston communities, ending with a plea for residents of the city to stay active in the fight against violence, ad-
mitting that "the police cannot do it alone." He spoke only
briefly before deferring to several young ministers, who took
the podium and exhorted the small but growing crowd of professionals to "take back our streets and protect our families
from the creeping menace of drugs and violence."

The housing agency director then introduced the Reverend
Nelly Yarborough. As she stepped to the podium, I took in the
familiar African American woman, neatly dressed in a skirt suit
and wearing beaded rimmed glasses. This caring older woman
had been a patient of mine for several years when I had a large
primary care practice. I always enjoyed seeing her speak; inevitably, her gentle voice would transform into that of a boom-
ing black preacher at the appropriate moments.

She began to quietly address the crowd, but her passion grew
as she began to quote scripture about the capacity of the love of
God to cover us all. Her voice was stern and gentle at the same
time. Her cadence began to quicken, and the pitch of her voice
began to rise; after a few minutes she was urging the crowd, at
the very limit of her voice, to "pray that God will save the gen-
eration of young people who seem so determined to hurt and
kill each other." She called for the group to pray, and the row of
ministers and officials behind her cried, "Amen!" and "Tell it,
Pastor!" When the Reverend Yarborough told the group to join
hands, all quickly obeyed, lowering their heads as she led the
group in prayer.

Families wheeled little ones past in strollers, curious about
the gathering of hand-holding business professionals. They
sauntered along, distracted in the way a minor automobile col-
lision only briefly slows the passage of traffic. After the spirited
prayer, the Reverend Yarborough stepped back from the podium and the housing agency director closed the program with
her own plea to "make a difference." Slowly, people in the
crowd began to hug and connect with one another, allowing

the seriousness of the preceding hour to give way to the relief of fellowship. The sun continued to peek through the leaves of the trees as the crowd began to dissipate.

I said goodbye to my colleagues and began to retrace the path of my morning run back in the direction of my house. Off to the right, I could see just a hint of the bear cages, mostly obscured from view by the trees full of summer leaves. I reached the corner of Walnut and Seaver and waited for the light to change. A blue Toyota Camry honked its horn and pulled up in front of me. As I peered through the tinted windows, I realized it was Roy.

"Hey, where you going, man?"

"Back home," I told him. "Just came from that vigil in the park."

"Oh yeah? How was it?"

"It was fine," I said. "People are worried, and they want to do something." Roy nodded but seemed unimpressed.

"Get in," he said. "I'll drive you home."

I did not have more than three or four blocks to walk, but I gladly took the opportunity to ride with Roy. Roy was settling in nicely to his new job at the Health Commission, and I was proud to watch the work he was doing.

Several months earlier, after many years of working in the senator's office, Roy began to think about leaving, just as the runup to the 2004 presidential election season began. After months of debate, and at my urging, he became a case manager as part of a new program at the Health Commission designed to reach out to young men who had been injured and who were getting ready to leave the hospital. Since I was the medical director and had fought for the dollars to fund the program, I took some of the credit for Roy's decision to join us. I had gotten the sense that after years in the senator's office, the job had gotten stale for Roy. Even more, his financial struggles had worsened as his sons and daughters grew older and their needs increased.

Roy had rejected the idea that he should be thinking about a career path and continued to resist getting himself in any position that would cast him as a role model. "I would be happy just digging ditches," he would tell me over and over again. I understood what he was trying to say, but I didn't entirely buy it. In his years at the senator's office, Roy had risen from office assistant to administrator of the office's local area computer network. He had taught himself to manage the computer network; his own inner competitive nature drove him to take on such challenges. But without the formal training and certification needed to show these skills, he knew that he could never expect the salaries that bona fide IT professionals earn. Eventually Roy would become the senator's Massachusetts office manager, but it was clear to him he could go no further.

I encouraged Roy to make a move that would allow him to share his life experience directly with young men like himself. The new program at the Health Commission to work with injured young men looked to be the perfect match. Within days of his being hired, it became obvious that Roy was especially suited to be a case manager. For one thing, Roy seemed to know, either directly or indirectly, most of the young men he encountered in the hospital beds on the surgical ward. I watched several times as Roy met a young patient and then looked him up and down. Then Roy would inevitably say, "I know you. Aren't you C.J.'s brother?" Or "Aren't you a Claiborne?"

"Yeah," the young patient would answer, at first wary. Roy would then smoothly explain where he fit into the young man's web of family or friends. The process was fascinating to watch, particularly as it violated many of the boundaries of self-disclosure and familiarity that most doctors learn during medical school and residency. But this was a natural and necessary step to connecting with these men. Once Roy could place himself in the young patient's world, the rapport was immediate. It was making a sort of cultural connection, the same type that I felt in my youth when an older church member would say to me, "Aren't you Fred and Jessie's son?" These were not asked as questions but were presented as statements of fact, spoken just so I would know that *they* knew. It was much the same for Roy. He wanted them to know that in a sense he knew them, because in some ways, he was them. And this connection proved to be a very powerful force.

■ ■ ■

Roy spun up around and then down Humboldt Avenue and then turned on Townsend before swinging onto my street. He pulled several doors past my house into an empty parking space. We sat with the engine running for a moment.

"Bet all those people didn't know that somebody got shot this afternoon," Roy said.

"No. Where?"

"Up in Dorchester. Two kids got shot. One of them died. They took him to City."

"That's crazy. What's going on in this city?" I wondered aloud.

"It's these young kids, man. Some of these young kids actually scare *me*," Roy said.

"They scare *you*?"

"Yeah man. Because if one of 'em gets a big enough battery put in his back, ain't no stoppin' him. You might really have to hurt one of these young kids."

"Don't say that."

"I'm saying, at least when I was shooting at people, everybody else knew what that shit was about. Nobody understands these kids' reasons, not even the kids." Just then, a lanky young African American man strolled by on the other side of the street. He was dressed in basketball shoes and khaki cargo pants. He wore an oversized white T-shirt that hung almost to his knees.

"See that guy?" Roy asked. "You know why he's wearing white?"

"No. Tell me."

"He is wearing white to say 'Right now, I ain't representing shit!' If he came out today with red on, somebody might think he was reppin' that Blood shit. Or if he was walking around with a Cowboys cap, then he might be Crippin'. So that ain't just a white shirt.

"He's wearing white so that he can announce to the world that he's not down with a gang or any kind of crew. And even if he is in a gang, he ain't reppin' his gang right now. He's just chillin'. Or he might just be showing respect to a hood he ain't from by not rocking his colors or tags in their hood. It's kind of like he's waving a neutral flag. That's what I'm talking about."

"See, none of this is like it was when I was growing up. I never had to think about things like that," I said.

"It's kind of the same for me. You wanna know the difference between my era and this era?" Roy quizzed.

"What?"

"Only certain cats were gangsters when I was growing up. And they were a different kind of gangster. It was a much smaller crowd, and they were clearly different from everybody else. Now anybody and everybody's a thug, and it shouldn't be that way."

"It shouldn't be any kind of way," I said, unsure where all this was leading.

"Naw, I'm serious! All you gotta do is look at the shooters. The aggressive kids back in the day were usually extremely bright, mature beyond their years, and easily identifiable as leaders or villains in any crowd they were in. Think about it: The kids that crash nowadays are just kids. Nothing unusual or out of the ordinary about any of them. Regular kids. That's what's scary. It ain't just the kids who remind you of Damien in that *Omen* flick anymore. It's every kid—even some of the good kids, too."

"That's what's frustrating," I said. "I know some young kids have guns just because they don't feel safe. Then there are other kids, like the ones you are talking about, who are mixed up in the gang life. And then there are kids like the one walking down the street wearing white who's just trying to stay out of it."

Roy shook his head. "But now more of these young kids are

getting mixed up in the gangbanging thug lifestyle because it's popular and recognized no matter where you go. So even the ones that used to get guns just for protection, now they're the ones all pumped up to use them. They don't realize it ain't a cartoon until they crash. They're so young, it's like a real life action adventure to them."

"So when you've got kids getting murdered by the dozen, a bunch of folks in suits standing around in the park holding hands just seems a little ridiculous," I said.

Roy laughed. "It does when you put it that way." His brow suddenly wrinkled into a serious frown. "You know, y'all have to stop thinking that you are going to totally do away with homicides. That's not gonna happen. You're not going to just stop all the killings. The way the streets are, there will always be situations where somebody gets into an argument or gets disrespected, and somebody gets killed. Then his people go after the people that did it and then somebody else is going to get killed. Some of this stuff you just can't stop. It has to play itself out. So the goal can't be *no killings*. Like if somebody hurt my daughter?" Roy puffed out a breath and swayed with anger at the thought. "Man, there ain't a damned thing you or nobody else could say to me about what I'm supposed to do about that without getting yourself in trouble. And it's not like there's some police intelligence system that could catch something like that. Too spontaneous. So the goal has to be this: Stop the violence and killings that you can realistically impact, and help the kids you *know* you can get to. Like the kids I see in the hospital."

This was a sobering thought, but I took it as a small helping of Roy's street-honed wisdom. I had learned by now that it was best for me to take the time to digest Roy's ideas and not react to them in the moment. Most often, as it turned out, they proved wise and unsettling.

The light was fading, so I invited Roy in so that we could finish talking inside. I pointed Roy to the living room and went to the kitchen to grab some snacks. I poured white pistachios into a ceramic dish and grabbed a bottle of Lambrusco from the fridge and two glasses.

We sat in the living room, Roy in the big beige easy chair and I on the couch. We were both hungry by then, and we each pulled large handfuls of white pistachios from the bowl and split them with our fingers. I poured us glasses of the dark sweet wine. We sipped it, and its effervescence cut cleanly through the saltiness of the nuts.

Roy was in a different place now. He had three children with a woman from whom he had had a nasty breakup about a year earlier. There were some things about the breakup that added to Roy's already aggressive edge, a bitterness that was clearly unhealthy and oddly concerning. It was an understatement to say that Roy was upset. He had been crushed by it. Only, for Roy, hurt always translated to anger. In fact, it occurred to me that Roy often found a kind of indignant anger as a response to many emotional threats and many different types of disloyalty.

I realized again, sitting here across from him, just how badly Roy had been damaged by the breakup. When I thought back to all of the conversations we'd had and the small fragments of painful detail he had dropped over the years, it made sense. This was the ruin of everything he had ever fought for. Roy's kids were his excuse for everything. They were his reason. He told me once that the breakup felt as if "one day somebody else decided I wasn't entitled to a family anymore, and nothing I'd ever done, good or gangster, could stop it."

As he related: "You know, man, that shit messed me up. The only way to describe it is like somebody telling a five-star general who's been in every major war over the last 20 years and got the war wounds and all, that his country doesn't want his services anymore. So you know what I did? I just decided to pick up and go. I was on some cross-country troublemaker shit. I got on a plane and flew out to South Central L.A. I always wanted to go there. And I just stood out on a corner, had some weed with me, took out a blunt and started smoking it, right there on the corner. I wasn't wearing colors or anything, so no-body thought I was a gang member. After a while some dudes came around like 'Who are you?'

"So I was like, 'You don't know me, player. My name's Roy.'

"They was like, 'Where the fuck you from?'

"I said, 'I ain't from 'round here. I'm from Boston.'

"So they was like, 'What the hell you doin' up in here?'

"So I was like, 'Nigga, I'm just standing on the corner smok-ing this blunt.'

"So they was just like, 'Man, you crazier than a muthafucker! You know where the fuck you at? You ain't scared?'

"And I was like, 'Naw, I'm just going to every ill hood before I die. I ain't scared.'

"So we just kicked it. Stood there smokin' weed. That was it. I made some good friends out there. . . .'"

Roy raised the wine glass to his mouth and drew out a long sip of the fizzy liquid. He settled back into the soft beige chair and propped his leg on the ottoman. He reached forward and scooped another handful of the pistachios and lay back again, holding his hand out across the armrest, his palm cupped open with the dusty white nuts. He worked a pistachio from its shell with his teeth.

After a while, he resumed: "Couple weeks later, did it again. Always wanted to go to Chicago, see Cabrini Green. Went into the projects, same thing. No colors, just stood on the corner with my blunt. Dudes came up, asked what I was doin', why I was there. I told them I always wanted to see Cabrini Green. And they was like, 'Cool.' So we just smoked the blunt together. They was like, 'This nigga is crazy!' Did the same thing in Marcy Pro-jects in Brooklyn, Queensbridge in Queens, D.C., Virginia."

"Sounds dangerous," I said, stating the obvious.

Roy tilted his head to the side. "Yeah man, but then I didn't care. The way stuff had gone down, I had stopped caring about what happened to me at all. I think back then, I would have preferred a spectacular death than a long painful life."

■ ■ ■

The story weighed down on me. Roy always impressed me as such a fighter. But the passively suicidal tone of his voice showed me how deeply he had sunk into depression.

"I am sorry I didn't know about all that, Roy," I offered. Roy dismissed this expression of guilt with a wave of his hand.

"How could you know, man? That was when I was totally cut off from everybody. And I am not in that place now. I know I need to be here and present for my kids. But you asked me, so I was just putting it out there."

"Fair enough," I said, feeling rebuffed. "So tell me this: how are you making it now?"

Roy shook his head skeptically. "I'm not too sure, man. I think I'm all right, but I am really not too sure." He took another gulp of the wine and held the glass up to the light for a moment. "Like I tell you all the time. It's a hell of a lot harder being good than being bad. In a lot of ways, I was doing better then than I am now. Seems like every day something comes up. My kids need things for school, the car starts making some crazy noise or the brakes give out. Sometimes it is hard to make it on what I am bringing in.

"But I'm not going back to all that street chaos, trust me. Just like I tell my clients: It takes a whole lot more strength to get up every day and take myself into work than it ever did to be out on the corner, even though I was pulling in thousands of dollars or whatever."

As many times as I had heard Roy say this in the more than ten years that I had known him, I had never been more convinced of his resolve. Now it was not as though Roy was trying to convince himself that he had progressed. Now, it had become a part of his life story, and this story resonated with the young men who now flocked to him for counsel.

"Things are definitely better with my family, too," Roy added. "I was talking to my mom. She's doing good. She does these substance abuse workshops now. I hear about her all the time from people who have taken her class. It's funny. I was laughing with her about how she used to be back when I was a kid, and how good she's doing now. We just both had to laugh. Like mother, like son." Roy laughed.

Roy squinted to read the time off the cable box under the television. "It's 9 o'clock already. I gotta bounce out of here."

We both got up and walked to the door. "Thanks for the ride and the lessons," I told him. "You are always schooling me."

"Hey man, it goes both ways, ya know?" he responded.

We clasped hands and touched opposite shoulders in a ritual hug. He trotted down the stairs, and I followed behind. I waited on the porch as he slid into his Toyota and sped off down the street.

The summer air hung heavy, but a breeze softened the retreating heat. I could hear the distant voices of children a few blocks over. Their playful yells mingled with the rumbling of the leaves on the many trees that lined the short city block. No sirens, no chaos punctured these sounds. I stood for another moment to drink in the sweetly ordinary Roxbury night.

CONCLUSION

After sitting with these young patients and hearing their stories, I began to think differently about my own life and work as a doctor. My interest in hearing from these young men was sparked by the connection to them that I felt as a black man. It was because I felt connected to them that I felt the sting of the barbs directed at them and at black men in general.

Still, the world in which I grew up was far different from the one in which they lived. As I made my way through college, medical school, and residency, I too was unconsciously affected by the images of young black men portrayed on television and depicted in the newspaper. When I was most honest with myself, I could find in myself traces of the same stereotypes and implicit biases held by the rest of the world. These biases led me to believe that I knew more about the motivations and life circumstances of these patients than I actually did.

But within minutes of meeting young men like Roy, Kari, and Baron, these presumptions were challenged, and other early impressions melted away. No matter how menacing young people like Jimmy or Mark might have seemed from the vivid descriptions on the ambulance trip sheet or medical chart, each time that I sat face to face with them, whether in their homes or in a car on a Roxbury street or in the visiting room at a medium-security prison, I was reminded that they were more like me than I would ever have dared to admit.

I expected that along the way I would meet at least a few young sociopaths whose stated purpose in life was to wound and injure others and terrorize their communities. In truth, I have met few of these, if any. Yet as I moved from hospital to agency to community, I heard these young people talked about in ways that were more animal than human. Phrases like "endangered species" are easily applied to young black men without considering the unfortunate implication that they are a different "species." Even words like *beast* and *herd* show up with disturbing frequency in media references to men of color. As a result, even before we meet them, they appear in our minds with monstrous images attached to them.

The doctors and nurses and emergency medical staff who care for these patients are not monsters either. Sometimes the overwhelming volume of injured patients and the numbing pace of the emergency care routine can harden even the most sensitive providers to the individuality of each patient, especially in the urgency of the moment. We providers who attend to these young patients hold the same unconscious stereotypes as the rest of the world, but by definition, we are unaware. Most providers want to engage these young people. We not only want to treat their wounds, we also hope desperately that these young people will not reappear in the emergency department with another life-threatening injury. The frustration and emotions that the providers express can be a reflection of our own trauma, but sometimes they are indeed a reflection of the implicit biases that we hold. These biases are not unique to us; they are the same biases that the whole society holds. But we have a responsibility as providers to understand the biases we carry with us. More than this, we have a duty to monitor how these biases change us and those around us when we are faced with a stigmatized young patient who evokes all of the usual negative stereotypes. And we must hold each other accountable by challenging these deeply held ideas every time we interact with a patient.

It is impossible to hear these young men tell their stories and not hear the deeper scars of trauma in their lives. Jimmy and Kari spoke clearly about the addictions to crack cocaine that affected their mothers' lives and affected their capacity to care for their sons. Baron was torn away from his parents at an early age. David, Kari, Mark, and Jimmy all grew up without their fathers, who were locked up, addicted, or otherwise absent. Even Roy could talk about the trauma of spending a summer on the streets, forced to rely on the decrepit bear cages of the zoo for shelter. None of these young men offered their childhood adversity as an excuse. In fact, rarely did they connect these early family troubles to their later life struggles with school, the police, drugs, or life in general. So used to taking the blame for all the failings in their lives, they simply accepted the blame for the scarcity of resources in their neighborhoods and the bad outcomes that it brought them. They failed to see the connection. And they are not alone in this.

And yet there is a wealth of evidence that such early life traumas are a powerful predictor of future life difficulties. That some young men turn to drugs or to the streets after their violent injuries is understandable. It is even more understandable given the troubles that have scarred their lives. The expectation that these young people can and will just "deal with it" is naive. Even Roy, even with as much success as he has had, still must struggle daily, not only with the injuries of the past but also with the expectation that he is solely responsible for healing himself.

In the often hostile environments in which these young men live, trauma looms even larger. It drives their reactions and decisions and disrupts the normal supportive relationships that all of us depend on. In this same environment, there is great pressure to "be a man" and not acknowledge these traumas, lest they appear weak. The pressure not to be seen as weak piles on even more pressure to prove that they are strong. All of these pressures prime the pump for the cycle of violence.

As providers, our job is not so much to fix the cycle as to understand it and to recognize it as an underlying cause of the seemingly bad decisions that our young patients make. Some of those decisions, while incomprehensible to us, make abundant sense on the streets, where any show of weakness can lead to victimization. Our job is not so much to judge their actions as good or bad, sensible or senseless, as to hear from them and understand how and why they arrive in these perilous places. There is an important difference between explanation and excuse. In this book, I am not trying to provide an excuse for the actions young men might take to remain safe or to construct a functioning identity for themselves. Rather, by understanding the cycle of violence for the purposes of explaining it, we can, I believe, understand the larger roles that we can play as members of the same community. For these young men, the horizon of possibilities for the future is so narrow that they must use violence to be "somebody." This alone speaks to how profoundly we have failed them.

Because of all of these differences, I believe that we need a common language for discussing these problems that reflects a more human understanding. We cannot simply discard these young people and send them off to jail. At the same time, it does none of us any good to cast them as victims and rob them of all control or responsibility. Again, I lean on the wisdom of Dr. Sandra Bloom, who argues that rather than see these young people as sick or bad, we should understand that they are injured. Injury is familiar to us. We know that past injury puts one at risk for future injury. We know that injury requires healing and rehabilitation. But we also know that not only must the injured person play a role in his or her own healing, the community must also play its role in finding and fixing the source of the injury. And above all, as we seek to "do no harm," we as providers must commit to avoid making the injury worse in our well-meant attempts to treat it with moral judgments.

In times of disturbing violence, it is tempting to look for interventions and programs that work. We grasp at new projects. We believe that somehow it is our job to rescue these young people. While I believe in interventions, the deep complexity of these young men and the problems they face will frustrate us if we look for a single cure, a magic bullet. The danger of this focus on interventions is that they often address only changes that the victim should make. A fundamental assumption of these interventions is that the client, in this case the young man, needs to change or else suffer the consequences. And even then, they often appear as well-intentioned quick fixes that expect individuals to change without acknowledging or attending to the social environment that created these entrenched problems in the first place. Often such programs also ignore the role, either active or passive, that we interveners played in creating those problems, by ignoring the hostile environments in which these young people live and instead blaming them for the scars that they bear. Finally, when some of these young men appear to be unreachable because they are so deeply scarred, programs often discard them. This all-too-familiar rejection then further propels these men down a path of destruction.

It is often not the interventions themselves that bring change but rather the assumptions and beliefs on which they are built. "Interventions" and "programs" are often seen as a panacea to whatever public health or social problem we face. But not all interventions are equal in their approach to social justice.

I am by no means opposed to programmatic attempts to address the problems of these young men. The CLUB program with which I got involved in the early 1990s was a program where men of color served as mentors to young men of color in the inner city. Many of these young men had lived tough lives in poverty or were involved with the criminal justice system. But the strength of the program went beyond the programmatic elements of group meetings, GED preparation, and job development. Inherently, the program had a core that made it unique: a focus on developing mutually beneficial relationships between the mentors and mentees. Embedded in the program was the belief that each member of the dyad would grow through the relationship. Though the CLUB program is no longer in existence, this was a powerful idea.

Ultimately, I believe that if we want to make ourselves safe, if we want to end the high levels of violence affecting young black men, we must focus on *their* safety: the very people we have blamed for making the community unsafe. We are only as safe as they are. The same safety that we desire, they desire. If we believe that locking them up, brutalizing them in the homes where they live, in the streets where they walk, in hospitals where they seek care, will make us safer, we are sorely mistaken. But if we see our fates and our community as directly tied to them, then we will fight the free flow of firearms, oppose more brutal policing, advocate for greater opportunities for meaningful work, and engage them as full partners in both understanding and addressing the problems that grip the communities in which they live.

Albert Camus wrote that "a man with whom one cannot reason is a man to be feared." To the extent that we maintain the idea that these young men are unreasonable, we can fear them. But when we understand that out of their collective trauma and the conditions of the social environment in which they live there emerges an underlying logic of physical and emotional survival, it can change us. It changed me.

And that is perhaps the point. As difficult as it may seem, it is not their transformation that we must seek but ours. It is only when we are transformed to embrace the humanity and defend the dignity of these young men—whether we are physicians or nurses or police officers or district attorneys or teachers—that we will engage them as full partners in our efforts to bring about healing, hope, and change.

EPILOGUE

In 2005, after spending 21 years of my life in Boston, I moved to Philadelphia to take a position at the Drexel University School of Public Health. While I left behind many of the people and neighborhoods that helped me to understand trauma and violence, I was coming to a city where the problem of violence exists on an even greater scale. Almost every morning, the Philadelphia newspapers and television stations report on multiple violent deaths and injuries. The year after I arrived here, in 2006, there were 406 homicides and 2,004 shootings. Each day throughout the year, the newspaper kept a running total of the number of violent deaths. This constant reminder of the loss of life became a source of trauma to me and to everyone else in the city. More tragically, the cold enumeration of the dead completely obscured their humanity and the complexity of the circumstances that led to the tragedies.

In an effort to change the language about violence and trauma in the lives of young men, I have joined colleagues in medicine and public health to create the Center for Nonviolence and Social Justice at the Drexel University School of Public Health.

The mission of the center is to heal wounds in order to stop violence.

A special focus of our work is to pursue programs, research, policy, and training to address trauma and violence among young people in the inner city. The aspect of the work that we believe to be unique is the focus on the health effects of trauma and how these effects fuel the cycle of violence. The experiences my colleagues and I share have led us to the conclusion that we cannot separate the health of young people from the trauma and violence in their lives.

The flagship of the center is a program called Healing Hurt People, which was conceived and is directed by Dr. Theodore Corbin. Healing Hurt People is an emergency department–based program that exists to reach out to injured young people who find themselves in the emergency department at Hahnemann Hospital, a Level 1 trauma center in downtown Philadelphia. A trained social worker assesses the trauma of such young people as well as their risk for future violence. The patients are then paired with a community outreach worker, who helps them accomplish a range of basic needs—getting an identification card, enrolling in school, finding a job—while also connecting them with professionals who can help them deal with the trauma that they have been through. We believe this work to be essential. While we realize that this program alone will not deal with all of the violence that happens in the city, this work takes advantage of the critical moment of injury—the "wake-up call" moment that Kari and Roy described—to break the cycle of violence. In the end, we believe that this is work we cannot afford *not* to do.

We are not alone in this work. Across the country, colleagues in Oakland and Los Angeles, California; Chicago, Illinois; Cincinnati, Ohio; Milwaukee, Wisconsin; Baltimore, Maryland; and Boston, Massachusetts, have developed hospital-based programs to reach out to young people who have been scarred by violence. In Boston, as in Philadelphia, young men who were themselves once victims of violence are employed as outreach workers to help current victims avoid the downward spiral of trauma and violence.

Dr. Sandra Bloom, whose writings greatly influenced this book, helped to create our Center, and her Sanctuary Model has provided a framework for our pursuits. Because of her work, we focus on principles embodied in the acronym SELF—Safety, Managing Emotions, Dealing with Loss and Making a Future—not only for the young people we see but also for ourselves, as we work to create a healing and nonviolent workplace.

Roy now works as a senior youth development specialist at the Boston Public Health Commission. In essence, Roy helps at-risk young men—some victims of violence, some former convicts—to connect with the school, work, fatherhood programs, and healing resources in their communities. Roy is perfectly suited to the work. When not at work, Roy raises his five children, helping them navigate the perils of growing up in the inner city. His love and concern for them provides the primary purpose for his life.

I see Roy when I am in Boston. We sit and talk while sipping coffee at South Station or meet for a long lunch at the Olive Garden in the shopping center near the building where he works. Roy's stories about his life and work constantly remind me of the complexities of violence and trauma in the inner city. Roy's personal stories also give me hope that change is possible, though it often is painful and takes years. Roy tells me that he has been writing about his life—the experiences that shaped him. I encourage him in this, hoping that in the future, he will have the opportunity to share his story in his own words.

The Center's goal is to change the dialogue about violence, away from terms of blame and dehumanization and toward a language of injury and healing. We also hope that these collective voices will help the systems that serve these young men—health, juvenile justice, mental health, education—to recognize the central role of healing in helping young people to change. We are encouraged that such a shift can occur if we can link the voices of those most affected by violence with the emerging science of trauma and allow them all to speak clearly to us.

Acknowledgments

There are many people without whose inspiration, generosity, and faith this book would not have been written. Primary gratitude goes to the young men who shared their lives, stories, pain, and healing. I owe a special debt of gratitude to Roy Martin, who agreed to have his story told unmasked and who was a partner in the writing and editing of his story. I hope that in the near future, he will tell his own story with dignity in books, film, music, or even just in the courageous living of his own life.

My colleagues at the Center for Nonviolence and Social Justice at the Drexel University School of Public Health—Linda Rich, Sandy Bloom, Ted Corbin, Ann Wilson, John Gaines, Dionne Delgado—have taught me volumes about how trauma and adversity can affect the lives of our patients. Even more, they have shown me that it is possible to create a culture of nonviolence and healing. The Thomas Scattergood Foundation, the Claneil Foundation, the California Endowment, and the Philadelphia Department of Behavioral Health have made this work possible.

Several mentors, teachers, and colleagues invested selflessly in my early development as a researcher, and their input has been invaluable over the years. They include Elliot Mishler and Catherine Riessman, who "co-parented" me as a novice researcher in narrative methods. Members of the Narrative Study Group, who assemble each month in Elliot's living room in Cambridge, Massachusetts, provided a community of colleagues who care deeply about the power of stories. Tom Inui, Jacqueline Campbell, and Lois McCloskey taught me the essentials of qualitative research and ethnography. Elijah Anderson's writings and friendship have deepened my understanding of the "code of the street." David Stone helped to broaden my understanding of the philosophy of science; our early writing together helped to crystallize ideas about how injury drives the cycle of violence. Jonathan Woodson and Cil Weekes-Cabey and many other of my colleagues at the hospital shared the hope that we in medicine can play a role in helping these patients heal from violence. Courtney Grey was invaluable in gathering, organizing, and analyzing the data that formed the foundation of the research.

The work would not have been possible without funding support from Boston University, National Institute of Mental Health of the National Institutes of Health, and the W.K. Kellogg Foundation. I am also grateful to the John D. and Catherine T. MacArthur Foundation for the fellowship that has focused attention on the lives of these young men.

I am grateful to those who read the many versions of the book. John Auerbach and Corby Kummer generously read my clumsy early attempts and persisted in believing that the end result would turn out all right. Jean McGuire and Barbara Herbert were tireless in their encouragement. Ralph Reckley painstakingly read every page of the manuscript, and each of his pencil marks improved the final product. Others who generously read and commented on early manuscripts include Soloman Evans, Michael Yudell, Rodney Elliott, and Michael Collins.

Special thanks is due to Kathryn Deputat, whose clear and gentle coaching helped to loosen my tongue to create a finished manuscript. Jack Weatherford, a brilliant author in his own right, encouraged me to put pen to paper and to "just do it."

I am also deeply grateful to my editor at the Johns Hopkins University Press, who believed in the idea from the start and worked patiently with me every step of the way.

I must especially thank my family for standing by throughout the writing of this book: the moms, Jessie and Nora, and my siblings, my nieces, and my nephews. Last but not least, I thank my partner Ted for his patience, support, brilliance, and inspiration. His feedback improved every aspect of the book. Knowing him has transformed my life completely.

Note on Sources

Even the most personal and subjective account must have some underpinning in the world of reportage and analysis when it crosses the territory of social issues and public policy. I am indebted to the work of researchers and analysts in helping form the groundwork for my insights.

In grappling with what Roy and Jimmy were trying to tell me, I found Elijah Anderson's 1999 book *Code of the Street* immensely helpful. Anderson's book is eloquent on the subject of respect and how it protects young men in the inner city. As he writes, "In the inner city environment, respect on the street may be viewed as a form of social capital that is very valuable, especially when various other forms of capital have been denied or are unavailable. Not only is it protective; it often forms the core of the person's self esteem, particularly when alternative avenues of self-expression are closed or sensed to be." Anderson's observations on the "urban uniform," mentioned in chapter 5, appear in *Streetwise* (1992). On the "golden hour" mentioned in chapter 1, see E. Brooke Lerner and Ronald M. Moscati, "The Golden Hour: Scientific fact or medical 'urban legend'?" *Academic Emergency Medicine* (2001). On the role of post-traumatic stress disorder following war experiences or September 11, mentioned in chapter 6, the following two articles were very helpful: D. Vlahov, S. Galea, H. Resnick et al., "Increased use of cigarettes, alcohol, and marijuana among Manhattan, New York, residents after the September 11th terrorist attacks," *American Journal of Epidemiology* (2002); and J. Bremner, S. Southwick,

A. Darnell, and D. Charney, "Chronic PTSD in Vietnam combat veterans," *American Journal of Psychiatry* (1996). The quotation from Albert Camus in the conclusion comes from "Neither Victims nor Executioners," in *The Power of Nonviolence*, edited by Howard Zinn (2002). The nettlesome article by Mike Barnicle mentioned in chapter 1 appeared in the *Boston Globe* on October 7, 1993.

In the conclusion, I make reference to the profound impact that traumas have on a person's future health. The most provocative evidence comes from the Adverse Childhood Experiences Study (ACES) conducted by researchers Vincent Felitti and Robert Anda with funding from the Centers for Disease Control and Prevention. This landmark study firmly established that early childhood adversity affects the health of adults later in life. The researchers found that various forms of adversity, abuse, and violence before the age of 18 were associated with a range of problems and illnesses as an adult, including alcohol abuse, depression, illicit drug use, heart disease, intimate partner violence, multiple sexual partners, sexually transmitted diseases, and suicide attempts. The results of their study are published in V. J. Felitti et al., "Relationship of childhood abuse and household dysfunction to many of the leading causes of death in adults," The Adverse Childhood Experiences (ACE) Study, *American Journal of Preventive Medicine* (1998).